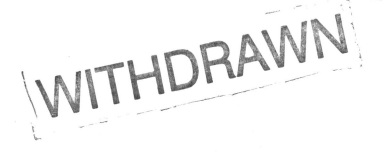

NOTES FOR PROFESSIONAL LIBRARIANS
AND LIBRARY USERS

This is an original book title published by Pharmaceutical Products Press®, an imprint of The Haworth Press, Inc. Unless otherwise noted in specific chapters with attribution, materials in this book have not been previously published elsewhere in any format or language.

CONSERVATION AND PRESERVATION NOTES

All books published by The Haworth Press, Inc. and its imprints are printed on certified pH neutral, acid free book grade paper. This paper meets the minimum requirements of American National Standard for Information Sciences-Permanence of Paper for Printed Material, ANSI Z39.48-1984.

Handbook
of Pharmaceutical
Biotechnology

PHARMACEUTICAL PRODUCTS PRESS
Pharmaceutical Sciences
Mickey C. Smith, PhD
Executive Editor

New, Recent, and Forthcoming Titles:

A Social History of the Minor Tranquilizers: The Quest for Small Comfort in the Age of Anxiety by Mickey C. Smith

Marketing Pharmaceutical Services: Patron Loyalty, Satisfaction, and Preferences edited by Harry A. Smith and Joel Coons

Nicotine Replacement: A Critical Evaluation edited by Ovide F. Pomerleau and Cynthia S. Pomerleau

Herbs of Choice: The Therapeutic Use of Phytomedicinals by Varro E. Tyler

Interpersonal Communication in Pharmaceutical Care by Helen Meldrum

Searching for Magic Bullets: Orphan Drugs, Consumer Activism, and Pharmaceutical Development by Lisa Ruby Basara and Michael Montagne

The Honest Herbal by Varro E. Tyler

Understanding the Pill: A Consumer's Guide to Oral Contraceptives by Greg Juhn

Pharmaceutical Chartbook, Second Edition edited by Abraham G. Hartzema and C. Daniel Mullins

The Handbook of Psychiatric Drug Therapy for Children and Adolescents by Karen A. Theesen

Children, Medicines, and Culture edited by Patricia J. Bush, Deanna J. Trakas, Emilio J. Sanz, Rolf L. Wirsing, Tuula Vaskilampi, and Alan Prout

Social and Behavioral Aspects of Pharmaceutical Care edited by Mickey C. Smith and Albert I. Wertheimer

Studies in Pharmaceutical Economics edited by Mickey C. Smith

Drugs of Natural Origin: Economic and Policy Aspects of Discovery, Development, and Marketing by Anthony Artuso

Pharmacy and the U.S. Health Care System, Second Edition edited by Jack E. Fincham and Albert I. Wertheimer

Medical Writing in Drug Development: A Practical Guide for Pharmaceutical Research by Robert J. Bonk

Pharmacy and the U.S. Health Care System, Second Edition edited by Jack E. Fincham and Albert I. Wertheimer

Improving the Quality of the Medication Use Process: Error Prevention and Reducing Adverse Drug Events edited by Alan Escovitz, Dev S. Pathak, and Philip J. Schneider

Access to Experimental Drugs in Terminal Illness: Ethical Issues by Udo Schuklenk

Herbal Medicinals: A Clinician's Guide by Lucinda Miller and Wallace J. Murray

Managed Care Pharmacy: Principles and Practice edited by Albert I. Wertheimer and Robert Navarro

Pharmacoeconomics in Perspective: A Primer on Research, Techniques, and Information by Robert J. Bonk

Global Competitiveness in the Pharmaceutical Industry: The Effect of National Regulatory, Economic, and Market Factors by Madhu Agrawal

Validation Instruments for Community Pharmacy: Pharmaceutical Care for the Third Millennium by Lilian M. Azzopardi

Pharmaceutical Marketing: Principles, Environment, and Practice by Mickey C. Smith, E. M. "Mick" Kolassa, Greg Perkins, and Bruce Siecker

Handbook of Pharmaceutical Biotechnology edited by Jay P. Rho and Stan G. Louie

Handbook of Pharmaceutical Biotechnology

Jay P. Rho, PharmD
Stan G. Louie, PharmD, PhD
Editors

Pharmaceutical Products Press®
An Imprint of The Haworth Press, Inc.
New York • London • Oxford

Published by

Pharmaceutical Products Press®, an imprint of The Haworth Press, Inc., 10 Alice Street, Binghamton, NY 13904-1580.

PUBLISHER'S NOTE
Medicine is an ever-changing science. As new research and clinical experience broaden our knowledge, changes in treatment and drug therapy are required. While many suggestions for drug usages are made herein, the book is intended for educational purposes only, and the author, editor, and publisher do not accept liability in the event of negative consequences incurred as a result of information presented in this book. We do not claim that this information is necessarily accurate by the rigid, scientific standard applied for medical proof, and therefore make no warranty, expressed or implied, with respect to the material herein contained. Therefore the patient is urged to check the product information sheet included in the package of each drug he or she plans to administer to be certain the protocol followed is not in conflict with the manufacturer's inserts. When a discrepancy arises between these inserts and information in this book, the physician is encouraged to use his or her best professional judgment.

Cover design by Lora Wiggins.

Library of Congress Cataloging-in-Publication Data

Handbook of pharmaceutical biotechnology / Jay P. Rho, Stan G. Louie, editors.
    p.   cm.
Includes bibliographical references and index.
ISBN 0-7890-0152-7 — ISBN 0-7890-1635-4 (pbk.)
    1. Pharmaceutical biotechnology—Handbooks, manuals, etc. I. Rho, Jay P. II. Louie, Stan G.

RS380 .H363 2002
615'.19—dc21

2001055478

CONTENTS

ABOUT THE EDITORS

Jay P. Rho, PharmD, is Associate Professor of Clinical Pharmacy, University of Southern California School of Pharmacy in Los Angeles, and Coordinator of Clinical Services, Department of Pharmaceutical Services, University of Southern California University Hospital in Los Angeles. Dr. Rho is a past recipient of the California Society of Health-System Pharmacists Practitioner Fellow Award, the Outstanding Preceptor of the Year Award for the University of the Pacific's School of Pharmacy, and is a two-time recipient of the Superior Performance Award from the West Los Angeles Medical Center's Department of Veterans Affairs. He is a widely published author and reviewer and currently serves as a journal reviewer for the *Journal of Pharmacy Technology, Formulary,* the *American Journal of Hospital Pharmacy,* and the *Annals of Pharmacotherapy.*

Stan G. Louie, PharmD, PhD, is Assistant Professor of Clinical Pharmacy, AIDS Research Unit of Los Angeles County AIDS Clinic, University of Southern California School of Pharmacy in Los Angeles. Dr. Louie is a past recipient of the Rho Chi Pharmaceutical Honor Society award and currently serves as a consultant to Bayer Biologicals, Syntex/Roche Pharmaceuticals, Oracle, Health Dimension, and Norman L. Yu and Company. His writings have appeared in a variety of publications, and he currently serves as editor for the *California Journal Health Systems, Pharmacotherapy,* the *American Journal of Hospital Pharmacist,* the *Journal of Drug Targeting,* and *OncoScope,* the newsletter of the Southern California Oncology Pharmacy Group.

CONTRIBUTORS

Cynthia Albert, PharmD, is Clinical Pharmacist, Scripps Hospital, San Diego, California.

Amir Aminimanizani, PharmD, is Assistant Professor of Clinical Pharmacy, School of Pharmacy, University of Southern California, Los Angeles, California.

Jennifer Cupo-Abbott, PharmD, is Assistant Professor of Clinical Pharmacy, School of Pharmacy, University of Southern California, Los Angeles, California.

Parul Patel, PharmD, is Resident, Pharmacy Practice, University of California at San Diego, San Diego, California.

Chapter 1

Introduction to Biotechnology

Stan G. Louie
Parul Patel

Biotechnology is defined as the use of tissue culture, living cells, or cellular enzymes to produce a defined product. The origins of biotechnology can be traced back thousands of years to a time when humans shifted from a life of nomadic hunting to one centered on perennial agriculture. These early biotechnologists discovered the ability to produce bread, cheese, and wines by adding yeast to crude mixtures of grain, fruits, and dairy products.

Although biotechnology has been used in food production for centuries, the application of biotechnology for the production of drugs did not occur until the late 1980s. The technological tools necessary to produce a recombinant drug required several scientific breakthroughs that were not discovered until the 1950s. The key scientific breakthrough that began the biotechnology cascade occurred with James Watson and Francis Crick's discovery in 1953 that deoxyribonucleic acid (DNA) comprised the blueprint for genetic replication and protein synthesis.[1]

Modern-day recombinant DNA technology exploits the machinery of a host cell to express the desired target protein. This technology has evolved with the discovery of two important enzymes: restriction endonuclease and DNA ligase. In 1973, Cohen and colleagues discovered that restriction enzymes and DNA ligase can be used to remove a DNA fragment from one source and attach the fragment to another source fragment in a cut-and-paste fashion, giving rise to the terminology *recombinant genes*.[2]

Restriction endonucleases are enzymes that cut at a distinct nucleotide sequence (motif) to produce well-defined DNA fragments called *restriction fragments*. These enzymes are capable of recognizing unique nucleotide sequences (recognition site) along the DNA complex. Normally, recognition sites are short and symmetrical sequences that are repeated on both strands of the DNA helix. When DNA is treated with restriction enzymes, either two blunt-end (even ends) or two uneven ends of DNA fragments result. DNA with uneven or "sticky ends" are cohesive because they do not have complementary base pairs. The ability to recognize and isolate a desired DNA sequence is now possible with the multitude of restriction endonucleases that are available. For example, the restriction enzyme *EcoRI*, derived from *Escherichia coli*, can recognize a nucleotide sequence consisting of CAATTC and its complement DNA.[3] *EcoRI* is then able to break the phosphodiester bonds between the G and A along this motif, producing two sticky ends of AATTC and CTTAA sequences. The staggered ends can be rejoined or annealed to complement bases by a DNA ligase, which catalyzes phosphodiester bond formation between two different DNA chains (Figure 1.1).

When a foreign DNA sequence is rejoined into a piece of cut DNA, the resultant product is called a vector, which is the essence behind recombinant DNA technology. Vectors are normally accessory chromosomes that have the nucleotide sequence required for replication and transcription when inserted into appropriate host cells. The most utilized vectors are bacterial plasmids, which are short, circular, extra-

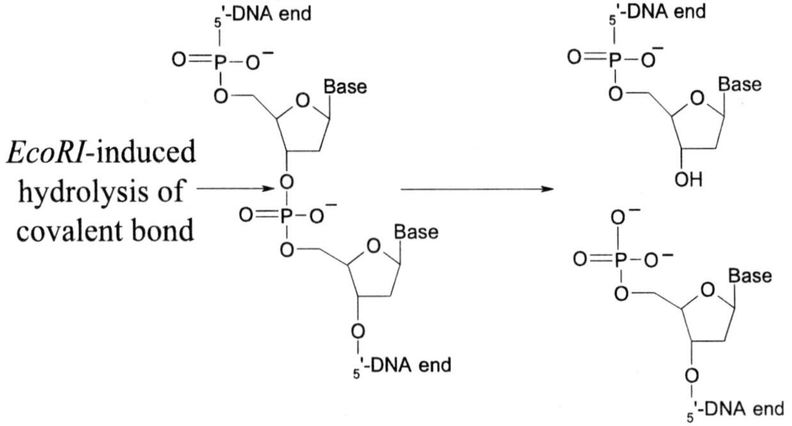

FIGURE 1.1. *EcoRI* is able to break the phosphodiester bonds between the G and A along this motif, resulting in two sticky ends with AATTC and CTTAA sequence.

chromosomal strands of DNA ranging two to hundreds of kilobases in length.[4]

Plasmids are able to replicate autonomously and are able to control their own replication (Figure 1.2). Every plasmid has a nucleotide sequence that includes an origin of replication *(ori),* and a nucleotide sequence coding for initiation factor(s).[5] Another important oligonucleotide sequence found in plasmids includes a promoter sequence that regulates the transcription of the gene.

Some plasmids carry genes that can inactivate antibiotics, which enables the host cells carrying the recombinant plasmid to survive in a medium or agar containing those agents.[5] The presence of anti-

Plasmid Insertion

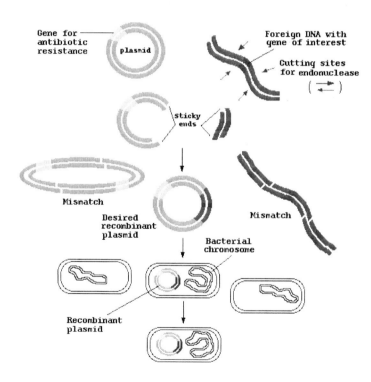

FIGURE 1.2. Production of recombinant plasmids

biotic-resistant genes will facilitate positive selection of host cells carrying the desired recombinant gene. One vector is pBR322, which is a bacterial plasmid that contains two genes conferring resistance against tetracycline and ampicillin.[4] In addition, pBR322 has recognition sites for restriction enzymes such as Hind III, Sal II, or Bam HI along the tetracycline-resistant gene.[6] Thus, a gene inserted along this sequence can inactivate tetracycline resistance; however, resistance toward ampicillin is retained. Therefore, the host cell containing the recombinant DNA is sensitive toward tetracycline, but resistant toward ampicillin. In contrast, cells that do not incorporate the recombinant vectors will not survive in a medium containing either tetracycline or ampicillin, whereas cells incorporating unmodified plasmids will be resistant to both antibiotics (Figure 1.3).

Newer plasmids no longer use antibiotic-resistant genes to select for host cells with recombinant plasmids.[7] Rather, the selection process utilizes plasmids which have genes that encode for enzymes, such as β-galactosidase. The *E. coli* gene *lacZ* encodes for β-galactosidase, which enables bacteria growing on agar containing X-gal to convert the colorless compound into an insoluble blue by-product. If a restriction fragment is inserted into the plasmid along the *lacZ* region, β-galactosidase activity will be inhibited, which is evident by the formation of colorless bacterial colonies.[5]

DELIVERY OF RECOMBINANT DNA INTO EXPRESSION VECTORS

Several methods can be used to deliver recombinant DNA into host or expression cells. These methods include microinjection, electroporation, calcium salt complexation, and viral transfection (delivery of recombinant DNA via viral infection).

Microinjection is a physical injection of recombinant DNA into the target cell, and is accomplished through the insertion of a glass micropipette into the nucleus to deliver the recombinant DNA product. The method is highly specific, but very inefficient because only one cell can be injected at a time. In addition, this method requires great precision because the procedure can cause cellular damage.

Electroporation increases permeability of the host cell by transducing electrical charges, thus increasing DNA uptake. When an electrical charge passes through a cell, it transiently creates holes

Cloning into a plasmid

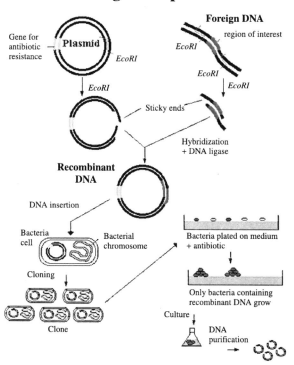

FIGURE 1.3. Cells that do not incorporate the recombinant vectors will be unable to survive in a medium containing either tetracycline or ampicillin, whereas cells incorporating unmodified plasmids will be resistant to both antibiotics.

within the plasma membrane and thus allows the DNA to enter without the help of endocytic vesicles. Other means of delivering recombinant DNA include the complexing of recombinant DNA with calcium salt (i.e., phosphate or chloride). When calcium salts are added to DNA sequences, they will form complex DNA and calcium salts. The addition of this complex into the culture medium containing the host cell will facilitate DNA uptake in rapidly dividing cells. Cells that are heated or heat shocked prior to the addition of complex DNA will facilitate intracellular uptake. This method is very easy to perform, but the efficiency is low because of cellular degradation of the modified vector. Methods using mutant bacteria have decreased DNA degradation. However, the major obstacle confronting this method is that only small DNA fragments can be inserted. Furthermore, some cells, such as lymphocytes, are resistant to transfection by calcium phosphate precipitation.

An alternative method of recombinant DNA insertion is transfection which is performed by injecting the host cell with a virus or bacteriophage containing the recombinant vector. Viruses and bacteriophages are able to penetrate cells with great efficiency. Unlike bacterial vectors, viruses can splice their own genome into the infected cells. In order for segments of complementary DNA (cDNA) to be cloned into a phage vector, it must have complementary single-stranded DNA restriction sites. The phage DNA can be cleaved using a restriction enzyme and the fragments are then purified. In order to splice the two DNA together, the isolated cDNA must have complementary single-stranded tails to the viral vector. This can be accomplished by blocking all internal restriction sites present within the cDNA. Synthetic oligonucleotide linkers are then added with the known restriction sequence using terminal transferase. The cDNA is then treated with the same restriction enzyme used on the viral or bacteriophage vector, thus producing complementary tails. The two DNA are then digested using DNA ligase. The recombinant DNA is added to lysates prepared from infected *E. coli*. The packaged phages are used to infect new cultures of *E. coli,* which then will incorporate into the newly infected host cells.[8]

HOST OR EXPRESSION CELLS

Several types of host or expression cells can be used to express the modified DNA plasmid. A majority of these host cells are prokaryotic cells. *Escherichia coli* is the most commonly utilized among the host cells, because it can replicate rapidly and is easy to maintain, since the medium required to maintain the transformed *E. coli* is relatively simple and inexpensive.[5]

Although bacteria are ideal hosts for DNA amplification and protein synthesis, prokaryotic hosts are unable to perform posttranslational modifications, such as signal sequence proteolysis and glycosylation. The major drawback of using prokaryotes is that cDNA is required to form functional protein, since prokaryotes such as *E. coli* lack the machinery required to excise introns (noncoding nucleotides).[5] Bacteria also lack the enzymes that are required to carry out posttranslational modification. This is important for glycoprotein, which may require glycosylation for biological activity. Furthermore, prokaryotic systems may be unable to secrete their proteins into the medium and hence the lysis of the organism is required to harvest the recombinant product. The lysis of the bacterial host may introduce contaminants, such as endotoxins, which may hinder the purification process and cause allergic reactions.

Yeasts, such as *Saccharomyces cervisiae,* have similar host properties as prokaryotes with rapid replication, but are more expensive to maintain in culture. *Saccharomyces cervisiae* has an advantage over prokaryotes in that it can excrete the produced protein into extracellular fluids. The secretion of protein will simplify protein isolation and eliminate the need to lyse host cells to harvest the desired protein. In addition, yeasts are able to perform posttranslational modifications, for example, protein glycosylation. This is especially important when glycosylation is required for biological activity, as is the case with erythropoietin.[5]

Both prokaryotes and yeast are limited in their ability to remove introns and form pre-mRNA. Thus, the transformed cells must have cDNA. Higher eukaryotic cells are able to remove introns and have the necessary enzymes for posttranslational modification. Examples of higher eukaryotic cells include the various mammalian host cells such as Chinese hamster ovary (CHO) and African green monkey kidney cells (COS).[5] The primary drawbacks of using a mammalian cell system include difficulty in maintaining cultures and the high cost associated with using this host system. Another drawback is that mammalian cells do not replicate as rapidly as prokaryotes and yeast cells.

DEVELOPMENT OF RECOMBINANT PROTEIN

For biological agents such as enzymes, hormones, or cytokines to have potential clinical applications, they must be produced in sufficient quantities to allow extensive testing during clinical trials. Large-scale isolation of the naturally occurring product can be cumbersome and expensive. Recombinant technology, however, allows the production of large quantities of the biological agent in a cost-efficient manner.

The first step is to purify the desired biological agent to homogeneity (single purified product). The purified protein is then enzymatically cleaved into smaller fragments, so that amino acid sequences from the peptide fragments are easily obtained. After obtaining a sequence of the polypeptide, a series of oligonucleotides are constructed to match the polypeptide sequence. Alternatively, the purified protein or peptide can be blotted onto a polyvinylidene difluoride (PVDF) membrane, and the NH_2-terminal residues can be sequenced using an automated Edman sequencer.[9]

After obtaining an amino acid sequence, a number of corresponding oligonucleotides are produced. There is degeneration in the oligonucleotide (also known as the "wobble effect"), in which more than one combination encodes for the same amino acid. Therefore, to ensure that the correct code is represented, a series of ambiguous or degenerate oligonucleotides are generated. The cloned cDNA is amplified using polymerase chain reaction (PCR) and is used as a probe to screen for a plasmid library which is complementary to the generated cDNA.[10]

The second step is to produce a complete DNA genomic library (Figure 1.4). The genomic DNA is digested with the same restriction enzyme as the cloning vectors, then the recombinant DNA is inserted

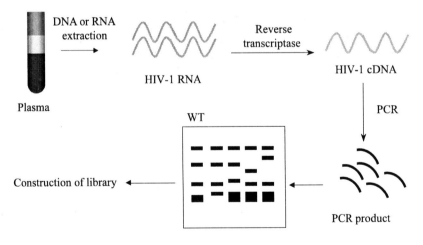

FIGURE 1.4. Production of a DNA genomic library

into host cells and propagated. The host cell containing the recombinant vectors will produce resistance to antibiotics in the agar.

Sometimes, it is preferable to construct a DNA library using RNA as the template. cDNA can be made using reverse transcriptase.[10] The cDNA is then linked with an expression vector similar to that used for genomic DNA. The cDNA library has a unique advantage since it represents only the coding region of the gene.

The library of DNA can be screened for the specific gene by hybridizing bacterial cDNA or synthetic oligonucleotides. The host cells are spread over growth medium, which results in the formation of colonies. Alternatively, viral vectors can be used by transfecting bacterial suspensions. The transfected bacteria are spread onto a culture plate and allowed to grow. A lawn of bacteria will form within a few days. The presence of clear areas or plaques represents viral-induced bacterial lysis. Each of the host cell colonies or viral plaques represents a specific DNA fragment of the foreign DNA. To determine which colony is expressing the DNA fragment, the colonies must be screened.

Screening can be accomplished by replicating a mirror image of the petri dish by placing a sterile nylon or nitrocellulose membrane onto the surface of the culture. The bacteria or virus will adhere to the membrane. The membrane is then denatured to immobilize the DNA. Once immobilized onto the membrane, radiolabeled degenerative oligonucleotides are added into a solution that will permit the binding of complementary nucleotide sequences also called "hybridization." Colonies or plaques that are radioactive indicate that complementary nucleotide sequences are being expressed. Colonies with strong radioactive signals can be further screened if an antibody directed against the protein is available or a biological assay, such as testing for enzyme activity, is possible. The host cells with the desired gene or nucleotide sequence are then grown to express the protein in large quantities.[11]

HYBRIDOMA TECHNOLOGY

As recombinant technology was being refined into a science, it was discovered that immortalized plasma cells could produce one distinctive type of antibody or monoclonal antibody. When an antigen or immunogen is injected into an animal for the purpose of producing antibodies directed against the antigen, millions of antibodies are produced. These antibodies recognize different regions or epitopes of the immunogen. The introduction of an immunogen will elicit the formation of B-lymphocytes to produce different types of antibodies, thus giving rise to the term *polyclonal*. Polyclonal antibodies consist of heterogeneous antibodies recognizing different epitopes on the antigen. Antibodies are derived from various clones of B-lymphocytes primed to different regions of the antigen, in which one B-cell clone will produce only one specific antibody directed to a single specific epitope.[12]

In 1975, Köhler and Milstein described a technique for the production of monoclonal antibodies.[12] Monoclonal antibodies are produced from a single B-lymphocyte clone, instead of a number of clones as seen in polyclonal antibodies. This is possible by immortalizing the B-lymphocyte, which can be maintained in culture flasks. Unlike polyclonal antibodies, monoclonal antibodies recognize only one antigenic determinant, which is homogeneous and specific.

The production of monoclonal antibodies can be accomplished by the fusion of two different cells, a primed B-lymphocyte and a multiple myeloma cell.[12] A multiple myeloma cell is a plasmacytoma or malignant B-lymphocyte, which is capable of producing large amounts of one specific type of antibody. The fusion of an immortal myeloma cell with a mortal plasma cell (primed B-lymphocyte) from the spleen of immunized mice will form a hybrid cell called hybridoma. Hybridoma is able to form a large quantity of homogenous antibody or monoclonal antibody such as the myeloma cells. Thus, hybridoma technology uses the machinery of the plasmacytoma; however, it is the primed B-lymphocyte which determines the type of antibody.

Köhler and Milstein used polyethylene glycol as the fusing reagent, which made the cellular membranes sticky and promoted the fusion of the two cellular membranes. Following the fusion of a B-lymphocyte and plasmacytoma, the cellular mixture is then cultured in a medium containing hypoxanthine, aminopterin, and thymidine (HAT). Only the fused plasmacytoma and B-lymphocyte will proliferate in this medium, thus eliminating the fusion of either two B-lymphocytes or two plasmacytomas (Figure 1.5).[12]

The hybridomas are then screened for the desired antibodies. Methods for screening include Western blots, binding assays, and enzyme inhibition assays. The selected clones are then subcloned three times to ensure the monoclonality of the hybridoma. These hybrid-

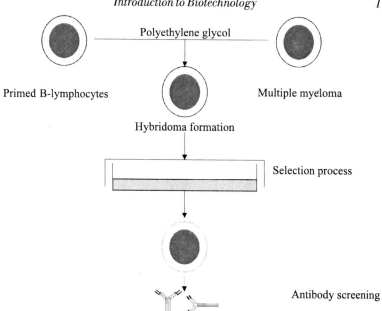

FIGURE 1.5. Monoclonal antibody production

omas are grown in a defined medium to ensure that the culture is free of both cellular and protein contaminants.

Large amounts of monoclonal antibodies can be obtained by injecting the hybridomas into the peritoneal cavity of appropriate recipient mice. The hybridoma will thrive in the ascitic fluid and produce large amounts of monoclonal antibodies.[12] The antibodies can be harvested from either cultured medium or ascitic fluid, and easily purified using a hydroxyapatite column.

Clinical application of monoclonal antibodies includes diagnostic test kits, antidotes, carriers for drugs and toxins, and means to eliminate targeted sites. Chapters 2 and 3 will provide a discussion of the clinical application of monoclonal and polyclonal antibodies, respectively.

CHIMERIZATION PROCESS

Monoclonal antibodies (Mab) derived from animal sources, such as mice or rats, can elicit an immune response when administered in humans. To eliminate the formation of antibodies directed against animal-derived immunoglobulin, the chimerization process was developed.[13]

The chimerization process is an approach used to "humanize" antibodies produced in animals. This is one strategy to reduce the potential for an unwanted immune response while maintaining the therapeutic efficacy of these agents. The process involves removing an amino acid sequence recognized as foreign, such as the constant region (Fc), and replacing it with an Fc from a human immunoglobulin.[13]

Chimeric Mab production has been successful in several instances. One example utilizes a chimeric Mab (Mu-9) directed against colon-specific antigen p (CSAp).[14] Two variable gene segments from Mu-9, V_κ and V_H, were amplified using polymerase chain reaction and cloned. These genes were combined with genetic sequences encoding for human Fc, thus producing the chimeric antibody. Since the chimeric antibody failed to bind to CSAp, a cDNA library of Mu-9 hybridomas was constructed. Using a probe, clones that postively hybridized with the murine V_κ and V_H segments were selected to construct a second chimeric antibody. The second chimeric antibody bound to CSAp and was found to behave in a similar manner as the murine antibody (Figure 1.6).[3]

In another study, it was found that a chimeric antibody directed against the multidrug transporter P-glycoprotein was better than the parent mouse antibody.[15] These achievements have paved the way for research in the production of humanized monoclonal antibodies, single domain antibodies, fusion proteins, and bispecific fragments comprising a Fab (the part of an antibody molecule that contains the antigen-combining site, consisting of a light chain and part of the heavy chain) from an anti-CD3 monoclonal antibody and a Fab from an anti-P-glycoprotein.[4]

NOTES

1. Watson JD. Molecular structure of nucleic acids: A structure for deoxyribonucleic acid. *Nature* 1953;171:737-738.

2. Cohen SN, Chang AC, Boyer HW, Helling RB. Construction of biological functional bacterial plasmids in vitro. *Proc Natl Acad Sci* 1973;70:3240-3244.

3. Meselson M, Yuan R. DNA restriction enzymes from *E. coli*. Nature 1968;217:1110-1114.

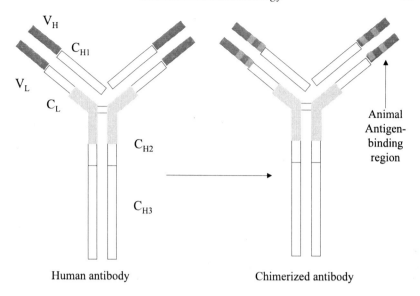

V_H

C_{H1}

V_L

C_L

C_{H2}

C_{H3}

Animal
Antigen-
binding
region

Human antibody

Chimerized antibody

FIGURE 1.6. Chimerization of antibodies

4. Sutcliffe G. Complete nucleotide sequence of the *E. coli* pBR322. *Cold Spring Harbor Symp Quant Biol* 1979;43:77-90.

5. Watson JD, Gilman M, Witkowski J. *Recombinant DNA,* Second edition. New York: Sci Am Books, 1992, pp. 13-30.

6. Smith HO, Wilcox KW. A restriction enzyme from *Hemophilus influenzae* I: Purification and general properties. *J Mol Biol* 1970;51:379-391.

7. Wu R, ed. *Recombinant DNA, methods in enzymology,* Volume 68. New York: Academic, 1980.

8. Bolivar F, Rodriguez RL, Greene PJ, Betlach MC, Heyneker HL, Boyer HW. Construction and characterization of new colony vehicles II: A multipurpose clone system. *Gene* 1977;2:95-113.

9. Khorana HG. Total synthesis of a gene. *Science* 1979;203:614-625.

10. Eisenstein BI. The polymerase chain reaction: A new method of using molecular genetics for medical diagnosis. *New Engl J Med* 1990;322:178-183.

11. Cochran BH, Zullo AC, Verma IM, Stiles CD. Expression of c-fos gene and of a fos-related gene is stimulated by platelet-derived growth factor. *Science* 1984; 226:1080-1082.

12. Köhler G, Milstein C. Continuous cultures of fused cells secreting antibody of predefined specificity. *Nature* 1975;256:495-497.

13. Waldmann H, Gilliland LK, Cobbold SP, Hale G. Immunotherapy. In Paul W. (Ed.), *Fundamental immunology,* Fourth edition. Philadelphia: Lippincott-Raven Publishers, 1999, pp. 1511-1533.

14. Krishnan IS, Hansen HJ, Losman MJ, et al. Chimerization of Mu-9: A colon-specific antigen p antibody reactive with gastrointestinal carcinomas. *Cancer* 1997;80(12 Suppl):2667-2674.

15. Panchagnula R, Dey CS. Monoclonal antibodies in drug targeting. *J Clin Pharm Therapeu* 1997;22(1):7-19.

Chapter 2

Monoclonal Antibodies

Cynthia Albert
Parul Patel
Jay P. Rho

INTRODUCTION

The fact that a monoclonal antibody (Mab) can target a specific antigen among millions of potential antigens has tremendous therapeutic value. Until recently, two major limitations associated with Mabs hindered their commercial use: (1) an inability to produce large quantities of antibody and (2) the immunogenicity of the nonhuman component. Both of these hurdles have been addressed with the discovery of hybridomas and the ability to "humanize" monoclonal antibodies, as reviewed in Chapter 1.[1] Hybridomas allow for the production of a limitless supply of antibodies, an attractive feature that has caused the number of Mabs in clinical trials to escalate. This chapter discusses the therapeutic use of Mabs as biological inhibitors, thus preventing the activation of other biological events that may lead to clinical sequelae.

ABCIXIMAB (Reopro®)

Introduction

Occlusion of coronary arteries can predispose a patient to myocardial infarction (MI). Reperfusion of these arteries is critical to prevent permanent ischemia and subsequent necrosis. Percutaneous transluminal coronary angioplasty (PTCA) is a procedure used to break up occlusions and help reperfuse myocardial cells. However, the procedure places patients at risk of tissue injury and possible reocclusion due to activation of adhesion molecules that bind onto the glycoprotein (GP) IIb/IIIa receptor (Figure 2.1).

GP IIb/IIIa is responsible for platelet adhesion and is active only after the platelet has been stimulated. Platelet aggregation is mediated by the GP IIb/IIIa receptor, a member of the integrin superfamily of membrane-bound adhesion molecules. Integrins are defined as subunit receptors composed of GP IIb and GP IIIa, which are capable of mediating adhesive interactions between cells or matrix. The GP IIb/IIIa domains responsible for binding adhesive proteins have been identified by their abilities to recognize the peptide sequence.

Coller described a murine Mab directed against the GP IIb/IIIa integrin receptor.[2] This antibody, now called abciximab or 7E3, exhibits a high affinity for the GP IIb/IIIa receptor. Abciximab binding prevents platelet adhesion, thus inhibiting activation of the coagulation cascade. This specificity makes 7E3 an attractive therapeutic agent for blocking adhesive proteins.[3,4,5] The binding of the 7E3 Mab onto GP IIb/IIIa has proved to be an effective antithrombotic agent, specifically in preventing arterial thrombi. To eliminate the binding

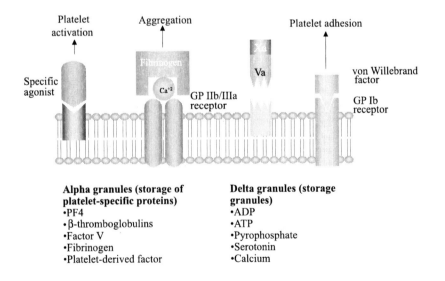

FIGURE 2.1. Glycoprotein-associated coagulation

of fibrinogen to activated platelets, large doses of 7E3 must be given to block GP IIb/IIIa receptor function.

Product Information

Abciximab is approved as an adjunct to percutaneous transluminal coronary angioplasty or atherectomy for the prevention of acute cardiac ischemic complications. It is also indicated in patients undergoing percutaneous coronary intervention and those with refractory unstable angina who are undergoing PTCA. These patients are at risk for abrupt closure of the coronary artery; approximately 9 percent of patients will encounter complications such as long-term reocclusion within six months after angioplasty.

Abciximab directly blocks the GP IIb/IIIa receptor, thus blocking platelet aggregation. Despite this fact, the use of abciximab as monotherapy has not been thoroughly investigated.

Pharmacology

Abciximab is the first in a class of glycoprotein IIb/IIIa inhibitors developed for clinical use as antiplatelet aggregation agents. Abciximab is a chimeric human-murine IgG1 Mab directed against GP IIb/IIIa receptor exhibiting potent antiplatelet aggregation activity (Figure 2.2). Abciximab is composed of an antigen-binding fragment (Fab) of Mab 7E3, which has been separated from the fragment crystallizable (Fc) portion, and replaced with a human Fc antibody. Removal of the murine Fc region reduces the potential for complement activation.

Pharmacokinetics

After intravenous administration of abciximab, a biphasic elimination is observed. The initial phase half-life is less than ten minutes, while the second phase half-life is approximately 30 minutes. In circulation, abciximab is bound to platelet GP IIb/IIIa receptors for ten days; however, platelet function recovers in 48 hours.

Abciximab inhibits platelet function in a dose-dependent manner. Ex vivo platelet aggregation studies demonstrated a blockade of over 80 percent of GP IIb/IIIa receptors at doses of 0.2 and 0.3 mg/kg. Platelet aggregation is not seen in response to 20 µM adenosine

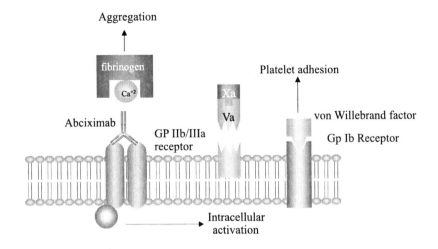

FIGURE 2.2. Mechanism for Abciximab

diphosphate (ADP), which translated into an increase in median bleeding time from five minutes at baseline to over 30 minutes at both doses.

Dosage and Administration

The recommended dose of abciximab is an intravenous (IV) bolus of 0.25 mg/kg administered 10 to 60 minutes before the start of PTCA, followed by a continuous IV infusion of 10 µg/min for 12 hours.

Clinical Trials

The EPIC trial was a multicenter, randomized, double-blind, placebo-controlled three-arm trial in which patients undergoing coronary balloon angioplasty or directional coronary atherectomy were at high risk for subsequent acute ischemic complications. High risk was defined as (1) acute myocardial infarction (MI) within 12 hours of symptom onset that necessitated direct or rescue angioplasty, (2) early postinfarction angina or unstable rest angina as defined by at least two episodes of angina associated with electrocardiographic changes despite medical therapy within 24 hours of the procedure, or (3) type B2 or C lesions with appropriate clinical characteristics.[6]

The EPIC trial is one of the largest studies conducted to date involving abciximab that showed a statistically significant reduction in the rate of composite end points such as death, nonfatal MI, unplanned coronary bypass graft, or unplanned PTCA for patients treated with abciximab compared with placebo (8.3 percent versus 12.8 percent).[6]

In another prospective double-blinded trial, 2,792 patients undergoing urgent or elective percutaneous coronary revascularization at 69 centers were randomly assigned to three regimens. The regimens were abciximab with standard-dose, weight-adjusted heparin (initial bolus of 100 IU/kg); abciximab with low-dose, weight-adjusted heparin (initial bolus of 70 IU/kg); or placebo with standard-dose, weight-adjusted heparin (initial bolus of 100 IU/kg). The primary efficacy end points were death as a result of any cause, MI, or urgent revascularization within 30 days of randomization.[7] Within 30 days, the composite event rate was 11.7 percent in the placebo group with standard-dose heparin; 5.2 percent in the abciximab group with low-dose heparin; and 5.4 percent in the abciximab group with standard-dose heparin (p value < 0.001).[7] Findings from this study suggest that inhibition of the platelet GP IIb/IIIa receptor with abciximab, together with low-dose, weight-adjusted heparin, decreases the rate of the composite 30-day end point by 56 percent without an increase in the risk of major bleeding complications.[7]

Adverse Reactions

The primary complication with abciximab therapy is the risk of bleeding episodes, which can occur in up to 14 percent of coronary angioplasty patients. The risk of bleeding appears to be greater in small patients (especially those weighing less than 75 kg), elderly patients (over 65 years of age), patients with a history of previous gastrointestinal disease, and patients who have received recent thrombolytic therapy. Vascular access sites are noted to be the most frequent sites of bleeding in patients receiving abciximab. Other serious adverse effects include thrombocytopenia, cardiac arrhythmias, vascular disorders, and pulmonary edema. Human antichimeric antibody development appears in response to abciximab administration in approximately 6.5 percent of patients (Table 2.1).

TABLE 2.1. Adverse Effects Associated with Abciximab

System	Effect
Cardiovascular	Hypotension
	Bradycardia
Gastrointestinal	Nausea
	Vomiting
Hematological	Anemia
	Bleeding
	Leukocytosis
Immune-related	Human antichimeric antibody development (HACA)

Abciximab is contraindicated in patients with known hypersensitivity to any components of this product or in patients at increased risk of bleeding (e.g., recent gastrointestinal or genitourinary bleeding of any clinical significance, history of cerebrovascular accident [CVA] within two years, or CVA with a significant residual neurological deficit, bleeding diathesis, or thrombocytopenia).

MUROMONAB-CD3 (Orthoclone®)

Introduction

The immunological events associated with graft rejection vary depending on the type of graft. The mechanism behind allograft rejection has not been clearly delineated, but several hypotheses exist. One hypothesis suggests that host T-lymphocytes respond to the peptide epitopes found on the tissues of transplanted organs. The presence of foreign MHC (major histocompatibility complex) molecules will trigger a cascade of immune responses. Other hypotheses suggest that the host response is activated because of the large number of foreign MHC molecules rather than host MHC molecules linked on processed peptides presented by antigen presenting cells (APC) in lower frequencies.[8]

Although the mechanism of immune response is unclear, the pathology of allograft rejection has been investigated. Graft rejection starts when neutrophils, lymphocytes, and macrophages infiltrate into grafted tissues releasing cytokines promoting vaso-endothelium injury.[8] Resultant immune activation leads to more tissue destruction, hemorrhage, and death of the graft.

Alternatively, a phenomenon called graft versus host disease (GvHD) can occur in bone marrow transplant patients. In GvHD, the transplanted marrow attacks host tissues, in contrast to graft rejection, in which the host's immune system attacks the allograft. GvHD can also occur in certain immune disorders.

The consequence of GvHD on an individual varies depending on the degree of MHC or human leukocyte antigen (HLA) matching.[8] Differences in MHC class I molecules result in a wasting syndrome characterized by pancytopenia as shown to occur in bone marrow transplantation. These patients experience mucosal destruction of endothelial linings resulting in diarrhea, skin and soft tissue ulcers, and liver destruction.[8] However, if the difference lies with MHC class II molecules, these individuals experience immune stimulation and autoantibody formation, similar to the pathophysiology of systemic erythematosus lupus (SLE).[8] The current therapies to prevent graft rejection involve immunosuppression and radiation.

Product Information

Muromonab-CD3 (OKT3) is a murine-derived immunoglobulin (IgG2a) with a heavy chain and light chain and a molecular weight of 50 kD and 25 kD, respectively. OKT3 is directed against cell differentiation cluster 3 (CD3) found on the surface of human T-lymphocytes, which, when bound, functions as an immunosuppressant. Muromonab-CD3 is one of three antibodies used for the prevention of graft rejection.

Muromonab-CD3 is indicated for the treatment of acute allograft rejection in renal transplant patients and steroid-resistant acute allograft rejection in cardiac and hepatic transplant patients.

Pharmacology

OKT3 exerts its activity by binding to a glycoprotein (the 20-kdε side chain) on the CD3 complex found in active circulating T-cells (Figure 2.3). This interaction results in a transient activation of T-cells with the release of cytokines blocking T-cell proliferation and differ-

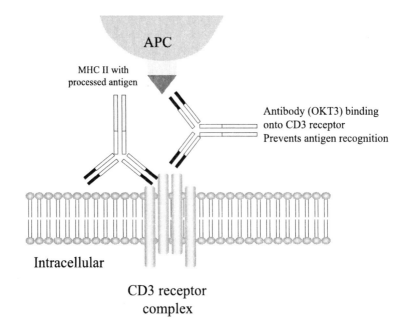

FIGURE 2.3. Mechanism of Action for Muromonab-CD3

entiation. As a consequence, nearly all functional T-cells are eliminated transiently from peripheral circulation.

Although the precise mechanisms by which OKT3 blocks the function of circulating T-cells is not completely understood, results of in vitro and in vivo studies indicate that the primary modes of action are (1) steric inhibition, (2) stimulation of T-cell activation and mitogenesis (induction of cytokine release), (3) peripheral T-cell opsonization and depletion, and (4) modulation of the CD3 complex.[9] OKT3 blocks the T-cell receptor (TcR) interaction with MHC class II antigens on the surface of APC.

OKT3 bound T-cells are phagocytized by macrophages found in the reticuloendothelial system, resulting in margination of T-cells into the intravascular spaces and redistribution to lymph nodes. T-cells are rapidly cleared from the peripheral circulation after IV administration of OKT3 and, therefore, are unavailable to recognize transplant antigens.[10] Finally, any remaining T-cells undergo T-cell receptor (TcR-CD3) modulation or internalization, during which TcRs with CD3 antigens are removed from the T-cell surfaces, rendering the T-cells CD3-negative and immunologically inactive.

Pharmacokinetics

After an intravenous dose of muromonab-CD3, symptoms of the cytokine release syndrome are observed within 30 to 60 minutes. Typical trough concentrations following a dose of 5 mg/day can range from 400 to 1,500 ng/mL. Similar trough concentrations of 600 to 1150 ng/mL are evident in renal transplant patients and are correlated with adequate CD3 modulation. Individual systemic clearance of OKT3 is dependent on (1) the total body load of available CD3 molecules, (2) rate of CD3 production, and (3) anti-OKT3 antibody titers. CD3+ cells in blood and lymphoid organs quickly consume doses of OKT3, resulting in almost undetectable drug serum levels after 12 hours. OKT3 elimination occurs slowly after the first dose with a half-life of 18 hours in the absence of anti-OKT3 antibodies.

Dosage and Administration

OKT3 is administered as an IV push over 20 to 40 seconds using a 0.22 μ filter. Adults and children over 12 years of age should receive a dose of 5 mg/day for 10 to 14 days. For children younger than 12, a dose of 0.1 mg/kg per day should be administered for 10 to 14 days. Some patients may require as much as 10 mg/d to achieve total peripheral T-cell depletion. Because no data are available on the compatibility of OKT3 with other IV substances, it should be transfused separately. If the IV line used to administer OKT3 also is being used to infuse other drugs or substances, the line should be flushed adequately with saline (20 mL) before and after infusion of OKT3.

Traditionally, the dosages of other immunosuppressive agents used in combination with OKT3 have been reduced or discontinued for the better part of the therapeutic course. This is done to minimize nephrotoxicity and excessive immunosuppression, but then resumed prior to the end of therapy. For example, cyclosporine or tacrolimus are commonly withheld until approximately day 10 of a 14-day or day 7 of a 10-day course of treatment.

Clinical Trials

Muromonab-CD3 is effective for induction of immunosuppression in patients receiving allograft transplants. In the treatment of acute allograft rejection in renal transplant patients, muromonab-CD3 is usually started at 5 mg/day intravenously for 10 to 14 days. A steroid, acetaminophen, and an antihistamine should be given as premedication before the first dose to decrease the incidence of initial reactions (cytokine release syndrome). Studies suggest that muromonab-CD3 is 68 to 95 percent effective in reversing rejection. Muromonab-CD3 is especially beneficial for patients experiencing renal failure induced by cyclosporine.

Muromonab-CD3 has also been shown to be effective in reversing acute cardiac and hepatic allograft rejection in patients who are unresponsive to high doses of steroids. Reversal rates in acute cardiac allograft rejection have been reported at 90 percent and 83 percent for hepatic allograft rejection. In addition, investigational trials have shown its effectiveness in pancreas and lung transplant rejection resistant to steroid or other therapy. However, when used for prophylaxis, it does not reduce the incidence of rejection or prolong graft survival. OKT3 has also been investigated for use in multiple sclerosis and psoriasis vulgaris, but has not received approval from the Food and Drug Administration (FDA) for these indications.

Adverse Reactions

OKT3 is associated with a wide spectrum of side effects, most of which are relatively minor. Most occur almost immediately after administration of the first dose, but some may occur days or weeks after injections. The adverse effects of OKT3 administration include diarrhea, nausea, vomiting, shortness of breath, dizziness, fainting, trembling, tachycardia (> 10 percent), headache, stiff neck, pulmonary edema (~ 5 percent), photophobia (1 to 5 percent), hypertension, hypotension, chest pain, and other miscellaneous effects such as pyrexia, fever, chills, itching, rash, hallucinations, tremor, aseptic meningitis, coma, and anaphylactic reactions (< 1 percent). The incidence of confusion and seizures is rare (Table 2.2).

Drug toxicities associated with muromonab-CD3 include serious, and occasionally fatal, immediate anaphylactic reactions. The reaction can be characterized by cardiovascular collapse, cardiopulmo-

TABLE 2.2. OKT3-Associated Adverse Effects

Frequency of Adverse Effects	Types of Adverse Events
>10 percent	Diarrhea, nausea, vomiting, shortness of breath, dizziness, fainting, trembling, tachycardia
5 percent	Headache, stiff neck, pulmonary edema
1-5 percent	Photophobia
<1 percent	Hypertension, hypotension, chest pain, pyrexia, fever, chills, itching, rash, hallucinations, tremors, aseptic meningitis, coma, anaphylactic reactions
Rare	Seizures, confusion

nary arrest, loss of consciousness, hypotension/shock, tachycardia, tingling, angioedema, airway obstruction, bronchospasm, dyspnea, urticaria, and pruritus. A similar reaction, often associated with the first dose, is the cytokine release syndrome (CRS).

Symptoms of CRS can range from mild, self-limited flulike illness to a severe, life-threatening shocklike reaction. Typical flulike symptoms include fever, chills, headaches, myalgia, nausea, vomiting, and diarrhea. The syndrome typically begins approximately 30 to 60 minutes after administration of a dose and may persist for several hours. Nearly all patients experience the cytokine release syndrome to some extent after the initial dose of OKT3. The severity of these effects ameliorates with subsequent doses. Severe reactions could include pulmonary edema, encephalopathy, aseptic meningitis, convulsions, or thrombosis of graft vessels.

The syndrome is observed after the induction and expression of pro-inflammatory cytokines, including tumor necrosis factor alpha (TNF-α), interferon gamma (IFN-γ), interleukin-2 (IL-2), and interleukin-6 (IL-6) after the initial dose. Suppression of the cytokine production may be accomplished by administering methylprednisolone 8 mg/kg injection 1 to 4 hours prior to the dose of OKT3. Larger doses of methylprednisolone do not result in better control of side effects.

Other toxicities associated with muromonab-CD3 include central nervous system-associated events such as seizures, encephalopathy, cerebral edema, headache, and aseptic meningitis. Due to immunosuppression, patients receiving OKT3 are more susceptible to bacte-

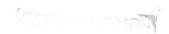

rial, viral, and fungal infections. Anti-infective prophylaxis may reduce the occurrence of infections.

BASILIXIMAB (Simulect®)

Introduction

Acute graft rejection occurs in approximately 30 to 50 percent of all renal transplant recipients, despite the availability of potent new immunosuppressive agents.[11] Although these episodes may be treated with high-dose steroids and OKT3, preventing an acute organ rejection would be more beneficial in terms of graft survival and health care costs.

As mentioned earlier, activated T-lymphocytes are important in acute allograft rejection. T-lymphocytes are stimulated through the expression of IL-2 receptor (IL-2R) that binds with high affinity onto IL-2. The IL-2R is composed of three transmembrane subunits: α (CD25), β (CD122), and γ (CD132).[12] Following IL-2 binding onto IL-2R, a number of intracellular signals are initiated, which ultimately results in T-lymphocyte activation as evident from the increased IL-2R or CD25 expression. The CD25 protein is the first and critical target in the up-regulation process.[13] Thus, a CD25 blockade will selectively inhibit only activated T-lymphocytes.

Immunosuppressive agents such as OKT3 and ATGAM bind onto the CD3 protein complex on T-lymphocytes, block antigen recognition, and cause a rapid disappearance of CD3+ T-cells from circulation.[9] These immunosuppressants are unable to differentiate between progenitor T-lymphocytes and activated T-lymphocytes, which can lead to lymphopenia, cytokine release syndrome, and increased risks of infections and lymphomas. By targeting only activated T-lymphocytes, the consequence of prolonged nonspecific immunosuppression is reduced. Mabs with the ability to block the interaction between IL-2 and its high affinity receptor would achieve more specific immunosuppression.[10]

Murine Mabs directed against the α subunit have been developed but are not suitable for use due to their rapid clearance. However, chimeric Mabs combining murine Fab regions with human Fc regions have the benefits of reduced immunogenicity, prolonged half-life, and enhanced effector function through the human Fc region. Two

Mabs, basiliximab (Simulect) and daclizumab (Zenapax), have been developed for use in preventing acute organ rejection in renal transplant patients. They are intended for use along with an immunosuppressive regimen that includes cyclosporine and corticosteroids (Box 2.1).

Product Information

Basiliximab is a chimeric Mab ($IgG_{1\kappa}$) produced by recombinant DNA technology that is specifically targeted against the α subunit of the IL-2R complex, also known as Tac antigen or CD25 of the IL-2 receptor IL-2R. Basiliximab can saturate IL-2 receptors on peripheral T-lymphocytes, inhibiting additional IL-2 binding.

Basiliximab is indicated for the prophylaxis of acute organ rejection in patients receiving renal transplantation when used as part of an immunosuppressive regimen that includes cyclosporine and corticosteroids. An advantage of basiliximab is a shorter, more simplified dose regimen that does not require outpatient administration.[13]

Pharmacokinetics

Basiliximab serum levels above 0.2 µg/ml are required to maintain complete and consistent blocking of IL-2Ra. Lower levels result in a reduction in IL-2Ra expression to pretherapy values within one to

---

BOX 2.1. Characteristics of Patients at Serious Risk of Complications Due to Cytokine Release Syndrome

- Have a body temperature greater than 37°C
- Hypersensitive to OKT3 or any other product of murine origin
- Have unstable angina or symptomatic ischemic heart disease
- Have had a recent myocardial infarction
- Are in uncompensated heart failure
- Are hypervolemic, hypovolemic, or uremic
- Are in pulmonary edema
- Have any form of chronic obstructive pulmonary disease
- Have a history of seizures or are predisposed to seizures
- Have cerebrovascular disease (large or small vessel)
- Have a disorder of the central nervous system (e.g., head trauma or a predisposition to seizures)

two weeks. Basiliximab preferentially binds to lymphocytes and macrophages/monocytes according to in vitro studies.

Single- and multiple-dose studies of basiliximab were conducted in adult renal transplantation patients. Cumulative doses ranging from 15 mg to 150 mg produced a median duration of IL-2R suppression for 35 days. A dose-proportional increase in C_{max} and AUC (area under the curve) was found at single doses up to 60 mg. The steady-state volume of distribution was found to be 8.6 L in adults. The terminal half-life is reported as 7.2 days. The elimination half-life does not appear to be influenced by age (20 to 69 years), gender, or race.

Dosage and Administration

Basiliximab is a sterile lyophilized powder that is available in 6 ml vials. Each vial contains 20 mg and should be reconstituted with 5 mL of sterile water for injection and further diluted to 50 mL total volume of 0.9 percent sodium chloride or 5 percent dextrose in water (D5W). Care should be taken to assure sterility of the prepared solution because the drug does not contain any antimicrobial preservative or bacteriostatic agents. Basiliximab lyophilized vials should be stored under refrigerated conditions (2°C to 8°C; 36°F to 46°F). Once reconstituted, the product should be used immediately but may be stored at 2°C to 8°C for 24 hours or at room temperature for four hours.[14]

Clinical Trials

A double-blind placebo-controlled phase III study involving 348 patients concurrently treated with cyclosporine microemulsion and corticosteroids was randomized to receive either basiliximab or placebo for renal transplant.[15] Basiliximab reduced the proportion of patients who experienced biopsy-confirmed acute rejection episodes by 28 percent compared to placebo. The safety profile for basiliximab was similar to placebo. Serious adverse events occurred in 54 percent of patients treated with basiliximab compared to 61 percent of patients treated with placebo. Overall incidences of infection were similar in the two treatment groups, 75 percent for basiliximab and 73 percent for placebo.

Another double-blind placebo-controlled study involved 333 patients who received dual immunosuppressive therapy with cyclosporine microemulsion and steroids and were randomized to receive either basiliximab or placebo for renal transplant. Basiliximab reduced the proportion of patients who experienced biopsy-confirmed acute rejection episodes six months after transplantation by 32 percent. Significantly fewer patients in the basiliximab group than in the placebo group had a steroid-resistant first-rejection episode that required antibody therapy. There was no evidence of cytokine release syndrome and the overall incidence of infection was no higher in the basiliximab group than in the placebo group.

A randomized, open-label prospective study was conducted in patients who received cadaveric liver allografts to determine the effects of ascites fluid and postoperative bleeding on the disposition of basiliximab.[16] One cohort received two doses of 20 mg basiliximab on days 0 and 4 and the second cohort received 40 mg basiliximab in smaller dose installments at more frequent intervals (four 10 mg doses on days 0, 2, 4, and 6). There were no pharmacokinetic or pharmacodynamic differences in the two dosing strategies, and receptor-saturating serum concentrations were easily achieved in liver transplant patients at well-tolerated doses.

Adverse Reactions

In clinical trials, basiliximab did not appear to add to the adverse events seen in organ transplantation patients as a consequence of their underlying disease and the concurrent administration of immunosuppressants and other medications. Basiliximab did not increase the incidence of serious adverse events compared to placebo. The most frequently reported adverse events were gastrointestinal disorders (75 percent of patients treated with basiliximab and 73 percent of patients treated with placebo).

DACLIZUMAB (Zenapax®)

Product Information

Daclizumab is a chimeric IgG1 Mab directed against the α subunit of the IL-2R. Daclizumab binds to lymphocytes expressing CD25 but does not activate them. Similar to basiliximab, daclizumab is considered an inhibitor of the IL-2 receptor. Both of these Mabs can inhibit the interaction of IL-2R and IL-2, thus blocking the mitogenic effects of IL-2.

Pharmacokinetics

Renal allograft patients were given a 1 mg/kg IV dose of daclizumab every 14 days for a total of five doses. Peak serum concentrations increased from a baseline trough level of 7.6 µg/mL to 21 µg/mL after the first dose to 32 µg/mL after the fifth dose. Data suggest that 5 to 10 µg/mL is necessary to saturate the Tac subunit of the IL-2 receptors to block activated T-lymphocyte response(s). Population pharmacokinetic analysis using a two-compartment model revealed a systemic clearance of 15 mL/hr, volume of central compartment of 2.5 L, and a volume of peripheral compartment of 3.4 L. The elimination half-life was 20 days, similar to the elimination half-life of human IgG of 18 to 23 days. Covariate analyses showed that no dosage adjustments based on age, race, gender, or degree of proteinuria are required for renal allograft patients. The estimated interpatient variabilities (percent coefficient of variation) in systemic clearance and central volume of distribution were 15 percent and 27 percent, respectively.

Dosage and Administration

The recommended adult regimen for the prophylaxis of acute organ rejection in patients receiving renal transplantation, when used as part of an immunosuppressive regimen that includes cyclosporine and corticosteroids, is two doses of 20 mg administered as an intravenous infusion over 20 to 30 minutes either peripherally or centrally. The first dose should be given within two hours prior to transplantation and the second dose four days after transplantation. For children ages 12 to 15 years, the same schedule should be followed, but each dose should be 12 mg/mm^2 (maximum 20 mg per dose).

Clinical Trials

Two phase III multicenter, double-blinded, placebo-controlled studies involving 535 patients receiving their first cadaveric renal transplants were performed to evaluate efficacy and safety. Daclizumab was administered every 14 days for a total of five doses and was given with either double (cyclosporine and prednisone) or triple (cyclosporine, prednisone, and azathioprine) therapy. Of these patients, 275 were enrolled in the double therapy and 260 were enrolled in the triple therapy.[17] Daclizumab resulted in a significant reduction in the incidence of biopsy-confirmed acute rejection during the six months and the year after transplantation (p value > 0.001) and a significantly lower dose of steroids were required as compared with placebo.[17] Daclizumab was not associated with any immediate side effects.

Adverse Reactions

In a randomized controlled clinical trial of renal allograft patients receiving cyclosporine and corticosteroids, daclizumab administration did not show any additional side effects or long-term consequences associated with over immunosuppression.[18] In addition, the incidence of posttransplant lymphomas did not increase by adding daclizumab to the therapy. However, there was a higher incidence of cellulitis and wound infections in the daclizumab-treated patients (8.4 percent) versus the placebo-treated group (4.1 percent). The most frequent adverse drug events reported were gastrointestinal disorders (Table 2.3).

RITUXIMAB (Rituxan®)

Product Information

Rituximab is a genetically engineered chimeric murine/human monoclonal antibody directed against the CD20 antigen (Anti-CD20 Mab) found on the surface of both normal and malignant lymphocytes (pre-B and mature B-lymphocytes). CD20 is expressed on more than 90 percent of B-cell lymphoma cells, but is not found on hematopoietic stem cells, pro-B-cells, normal plasma cells, or other normal tissues. It regulates the activation process for cell cycle initiation and differentiation. Rituximab is approved for the treatment of relapsed or refractory low-grade or follicular, CD20-positive, B-cell non-Hodgkin's lymphoma.

TABLE 2.3. Adverse Reactions Associated with Daclizumab

Organ Systems	Types of Adverse Events
Gastrointestinal	Constipation, nausea, diarrhea, vomiting, abdominal pain, pyrosis, dyspepsia, abdominal distention, epigastric pain not food related
Central nervous system/peripheral nervous system	Tremor, headache, dizziness
Urinary	Oliguria, dysuria, renal tubular necrosis
Respiratory	Dyspnea, pulmonary edema, cough
Skin	Impaired wound healing without infection, acne
Musculoskeletal	Back pain
Cardiac	Tachycardia
Hematologic	Thrombosis, bleeding, lymphocele
Autonomic nervous system	Hypertension, hypotension, aggravated hypertension
Psychiatric	Insomnia
General	Posttraumatic pain, chest pain, fever, pain, fatigue

Pharmacology

Anti-CD20 Mab is an $IgG_1\kappa$ containing a murine light- and heavy-chain variable or antigen-binding region. The antibody has been chimerized to express a human Fc region. Anti-CD20 binding onto the surface antigen will cause tumor cell death through several mechanisms. This includes complement-dependent cytotoxicity, where antibody binding will activate complement assembly to form cytotoxic pores in the membrane of target T-cells. In addition, anti-CD20 binding can recruit natural killer cells, which will then activate antibody-dependent cell-mediated cytotoxicity (ADCC). Another direct effect of anti-CD20 binding is the induction of cellular suicide or apoptosis where cell death is not cytotoxic. Rather, cells undergoing apoptosis will have activated endonuclease activities, thus causing DNA fragmentation.

Pharmacokinetics

Patients were given doses of 10, 50, 100, 250, or 500 mg/m^2 as an IV infusion, in which serum levels and the half-life of rituximab were proportional to dose. Pharmacokinetic analysis in patients receiving an intravenous dose of 100 mg/m^2 or greater demonstrated a mean serum half-life of 105.6 hours. In nine patients who were given 375 mg/m^2 as an IV infusion for four doses, the mean serum half-life was 59.8 hours (range 11.1 to 104.5 hours) after the first infusion and 174 hours (range 26 to 442 hours) after the fourth infusion. The peak and trough serum levels of rituximab were inversely correlated with baseline values for the number of circulating CD20-positive B-cells and measures of disease burden.

Dosage and Administration

Rituximab is usually administered (375 mg/m^2) as an IV infusion once weekly for four doses (days 1, 8, 15, and 22). Since hypersensitivity may occur, this product should not be administered as an intravenous push or bolus. Premedication that prevents hypersensitivity reactions consists of acetaminophen and diphenhydramine. Since transient hypotension may occur during rituximab infusion, withholding antihypertensive medications 12 hours prior to infusion should be considered.

First infusion: Administer rituximab at an initial rate of 50 mg/hr. If hypersensitivity does not occur, escalate the infusion rate in 50 mg/hr increments every 30 minutes, to a maximum of 400 mg/hr. If hypersensitivity or an infusion-related event develops, the infusion should be temporarily slowed or interrupted. The infusion can continue at one-half the previous rate upon improvement of patient symptoms.

Subsequent infusions: Administer at an initial rate of 100 mg/hr, and increase by 100 mg/hr increments at 30-minute intervals, to a maximum of 400 mg/hr as tolerated. Rituximab is stable for 24 hours at 2° to 8°C and 12 hours at room temperature. It is contraindicated in patients with known Type I hypersensitivity or anaphylactic reactions to murine proteins. Parameters requiring monitoring during rituximab therapy include complete blood counts, platelets, and blood pressure.

Adverse Reactions

Adverse event data were based on studies of lymphoma patients with bulky disease, as defined by lesions greater than 10 cm. Infusion-related symptoms of fever, chills, and rigor were experienced by a majority of patients (80 percent) following the first dose. Other adverse effects manifesting within two hours included nausea, urticaria, fatigue, headache, pruritus, bronchospasm, dyspnea, angioedema, rhinitis, vomiting, hypotension, flushing, and pain at disease sites (Table 2.4). These symptoms decreased in incidence (40 percent) upon subsequent infusions and were completely reversed upon initiation of supportive care.

Rituximab therapy resulted in B-cell depletion in 80 percent of patients, but it did not increase the incidence of infection overall. Serious infections which included bacteremia, polymicrobial sepsis, and herpes simplex infections were manifested in six (9 percent) patients. Severe neutropenia (1.9 percent), leukopenia, thrombocytopenia, and arrhythmias (1.3 percent each) were also reported as adverse effects. Patients receiving multiple courses of rituximab reported a similar incidence of adverse effects following the first infusion. Retreated patients complained of asthenia, throat irritation, flushing, tachycardia, and leukopenia more often following subsequent doses. For those patients with lesions greater

TABLE 2.4. Adverse Reactions Associated with Rituximab

System	Reaction
Whole body	• Flulike symptoms
	• Fevers
	• Chills
	• Asthenia
	• Headache
	• Myalgias
	• Arthralgias
Cardiovascular	• Hypotension
Digestive	• Nausea
	• Vomiting
Skin	• Pruritis
	• Rash
Respiratory	• Bronchospasm

than 10 cm in diameter, the most frequently reported adverse events were dizziness, neutropenia, thrombocytopenia, myalgia, anemia, and chest pain. Bulky diseased patients had a higher incidence of any grade 3 or 4 event (31 percent versus 13 percent) as compared to patients with lesions less than 10 cm in diameter.

TRASTUZUMAB (Herceptin®)

Introduction

Breast cancer is among the most commonly occurring cancers in women. Approximately 25 to 30 percent of patients with breast cancer have a genetic alteration in which there is an overexpression of the *HER2/neu* gene.[19] The *HER2* gene encodes for a receptor that is similar to the epidermal growth factor receptor. Tumors that overexpress this protein are usually more aggressive and resistant to chemotherapy. Clinically, overexpression of this gene carries a poor prognosis as measured by lower overall survival and disease-free survival.[20] Inhibition in ligand-receptor binding can reduce the rate of proliferation. Thus, antibodies directed against the receptor can inhibit the growth of tumors.

Product Information

Trastuzumab is a recombinant DNA-derived humanized murine/human anti-p185-*HER2* Mab. Trastuzumab selectively binds to the *HER2* receptor and inhibits cellular proliferation, especially the cells which overexpress this receptor.

Trastuzumab is available as a lyophilized powder containing 440 mg in each multidose vial and is stable at 2°C to 8°C before reconstitution until the expiration date. The powder should be reconstituted with 20 ml of bacteriostatic water for injection. The reconstituted multidose vial is stable for 28 days if placed back under refrigeration. Any remaining reconstituted doses should be discarded after 28 days. If sterile water for injection is used, the solution should be used immediately and any unused portion should be discarded. The 21 mg/mL concentration of trastuzumab should be diluted in 250 mL of 0.9 percent NaCl. Diluted trastuzumab is stable for up to 24 hours at room temperature, but it should be kept refrigerated until use. Trastuzumab should not be administered or mixed with dextrose solutions.

Pharmacokinetics

Pharmacokinetic data were derived from a study conducted on breast cancer patients with metastatic disease. Trastuzumab follows dose-dependent pharmacokinetics with short infusions of 10 to 500 mg given weekly. The volume of distribution was found to be approximately 44 mL/kg. The half-life increased from 1.7 days at the 10 mg dose to 12 days at 500 mg. The half-life was found to be intermediate of the aforementioned values (5.8 days) when patients were given a loading dose of 4 mg/kg followed by a weekly maintenance dose of 2 mg/kg. Steady-state peak and trough concentrations were 123 μg/mL and 79 μg/mL, respectively. When trastuzumab was administered concomitantly with paclitaxel, trough concentrations increased by 1.5-fold as compared to trough concentrations of trastuzumab combined with anthracycline and cyclophosphamide.

Dosage and Administration

Trastuzumab is indicated for the treatment of metastatic breast cancer with overexpression of *p185-HER2* receptor. The recommended dosing regimen begins with a loading dose of 4 mg/kg given as an intravenous infusion over 90 minutes. This is followed by a weekly infusion of 2 mg/kg given over 30 minutes, either as single therapy or in combination regimens of cytotoxic chemotherapy such as paclitaxel in patients who are treatment naive. It cannot be administered as an intravenous push or bolus.[20]

Clinical Trials

A phase II study of multiple-dose intravenous administration of trastuzumab in patients with metastatic breast cancer overly expressing *HER2* was performed in 46 patients. Patients received a loading dose of 250 mg of intravenous trastuzumab, followed by 100 mg given once weekly for ten weeks. Results revealed one complete remission and four partial remissions with an overall response rate of 11.6 percent. Trastuzumab was well tolerated with minimal toxicities that included fever and chills.

A phase II multicenter open-label study was conducted involving 39 breast cancer patients with overexpression of *HER2/neu* who were previously treated with conventional cytotoxic chemotherapy. These patients were given a combination of trastuzumab plus cisplatin. The intent of this study stemmed from data suggesting marked reduction in both size and number of carcinomas when Mab was combined with chemotherapy. In this study, patients received a loading dose of trastuzumab (250 mg IV) on day 0, followed by weekly doses of 100 mg IV for nine weeks and cisplatin (75 mg/m^2) on days 1, 29, and 57. Only 37 of the 39 patients enrolled could be evaluated in which ten patients (24 percent) had partial responses. There was no evidence of increased toxicity due to cisplatin when combined with trastuzumab. This study showed evidence of additive or synergistic activity when trastuzumab was used in combination with chemotherapy.[21]

Adverse Reactions

Trastuzumab is well tolerated; only flulike symptoms have been related to its administration.[22] Common infusion-related side effects with initial dose include chills, fever, headache, nausea, vomiting, and weakness. Other side effects include leukopenia, anemia, diarrhea, abdominal pain, and infections.

PALIVIZUMAB (Synagis®)

Introduction

Respiratory syncytial virus (RSV) is the leading cause of serious respiratory tract disease in infants and children.[23] The infection most often occurs in children from six weeks to two years of age but can also infect adults. Infections tend to be seasonal with peaks in the winter and rainy seasons.[24] Ribavirin is the only current effective treatment available, but its use is limited due to the requirement of prolonged aerosol administration and the exposure risk to pregnant women. Ideally, a vaccine against RSV infection would be the best form of prevention.

Passive immunization with RSV-IgIV (RespiGam), a polyclonal intravenous immunoglobulin discussed in Chapter 3, has shown efficacy as prophylaxis against RSV infections. However, widespread shortage and lengthy (approximately three hours) monthly intravenous infusions are some of the disadvantages associated with RSV-IgIV use.

Product Information

Palivizumab is a recombinant humanized Mab against the F protein of RSV. The F protein mediates fusion of the virus with cell membranes and subsequent cell-to-cell spread of the virus.[24] Preclinical studies have shown palivizumab to be 50 to 100 times more potent and concentrated than RespiGam.[25]

Palivizumab is indicated for the prophylaxis of RSV infection in infants and children who are at an increased risk for severe disease, especially those with chronic lung disease receiving medical management on a long-term basis.[26]

Pharmacokinetics

The pharmacokinetic profile of palivizumab is similar to a human IgG1 antibody in adults with a half-life of 18 days. In infants younger than 24 months of age, the reported half-life is 20 days. A 15 mg/kg intramuscular dose of palivizumab produced 30-day mean trough concentrations of 37 µg/mL after the first injection and 57 µg/mL, 68 µg/mL, and 72 µg/mL after the second through fourth injections, respectively.

Dosage and Administration

Palivizumab is administered intramuscularly (IM) in a dose of 15 mg/kg once a month during the RSV season (up to five doses). It does not interfere with vaccine administration. Palivizumab is available in 100 mg vials that must be used within six hours after opening. To minimize waste, physicians should administer doses to two or more eligible patients at the time of vial opening, if possible.

Clinical Trials

Impact-RSV was a multicenter, double-blind, randomized, placebo-controlled clinical trial of palivizumab involving 1,502 infants.

Subjects for the study included 24-month-old children with bronchopulmonary dysplasia (BPD) and premature infants at six months of age. At RSV season onset, five IM doses (15 mg/kg) of either palivizumab or placebo were given at 30-day intervals. RSV hospitalizations occurred in 4.8 percent (48/1002) patients in the palivizumab group as compared to 10.6 percent (53/500) with placebo. Overall, palivizumab administration showed a 55 percent reduction in RSV-related hospitalizations with no significant adverse effects. The development of pain and swelling at the injection site was comparable to placebo.[27]

Adverse Reactions

The adverse events associated with palivizumab administration were derived from the Impact-RSV trial. Only five participants discontinued use of palivizumab due to complaints of nausea and vomiting (2), erythema and other injection site reactions (1), and preexisting medical conditions requiring management (2). One death due to sudden infant death syndrome (SIDS) occurred in the palivizumab-treated group as compared to two deaths with placebo. The most commonly reported adverse effects were cough, wheeze, bronchiolitis, pneumonia, bronchitis, asthma, croup, dyspnea, sinusitis, apnea, and failure to thrive.

NOTES

1. Köhler G, Milstein C. Continuous cultures of fused cells secreting antibody of predefined specificity. *Nature* 1975;256:495-497.

2. Coller BS. A new murine monoclonal antibody reports an activation dependent change in the conformation and/or microenvironment of the glycoprotein IIb/IIIa complex. *J Clin Invest* 1985;76:101-108.

3. Coller BS, Folts JD, Smith SR, Scudder LE, Jordan R. Abolition of in vivo platelet thrombus formation in primates with monoclonal antibodies against the platelet glycoprotein IIb/IIIa receptor. *Circulation* 1989;80:1766-1774.

4. Bates ER, McGillem MJ, Mickelson JK, Pitt B, Mancini GB. A monoclonal antibody against the platelet glycoprotein IIb/IIIa receptor complex prevents aggregation and thrombosis in a canine model of coronary angioplasty. *Circulation* 1991;84:2463-2469.

5. Sudo Y, Lucchesi BR. Inhibition of platelet GPIIb/IIIa receptor with monoclonal antibody [7E3-F(abí)2] prevents arterial, but not venous rethrombosis [Abstract]. *Circulation* 1994;90(Suppl I):1-181.

6. EPIC Investigators. Use of a monoclonal antibody directed against the platelet glycoprotein IIb/IIIa receptor in high-risk coronary angioplasty. *N Engl J Med* 1994;330:956-961.

7. The EPILOG Investigators. Platelet glycoprotein IIb/IIIa receptor blockade and low-dose heparin during percutaneous coronary revascularization. *N Engl J Med* 1997;336:1689-1696.

8. Tizard IR. Organ transplantation. In *Immunology: An introduction,* Fourth edition. Philadelphia: Saunders College Publishing, 1995.

9. Anonymous. New monoclonal antibodies to prevent transplant rejection. *The Medical Letter on Drugs and Therapeutics* 1998;40:93-94.

10. Charpentier B, Thervet E. Placebo-controlled study of a humanized anti-TAC monoclonal antibody in dual therapy for prevention of acute rejection after renal transplantation. *Transplant Proc* 1998;30:1331-1332.

11. Matas AJ, Gillingham KJ, Payne WD, Najarian JS. The impact of an acute rejection episode on long-term renal allograft survival (t1/2). *Transplantation* 1994;57:857-859.

12. Leonard WJ, Depper JM, Crabtree GR, Rudikoff S, Pumphrey J, Robb RJ, Kronke M, Svetlik PB, Peffer NJ, Waldmann TA. Molecular cloning and expression of cDNAs for the human IL-2R. *Nature* 1984;311:626-631.

13. Kahan BD, Rajagopalan PR, Hall M. Reduction of the occurrence of acute cellular rejection among renal allograft recipients treated with basiliximab, a chimeric αIL-2R mAb. *Transplantation* 1999;67:276-284.

14. Product Information: Simulect, basiliximab. Novartis Pharmaceuticals, East Hanover, NJ, 1998.

15. Nashan B, Moore R, Amlot P, Schmidt A, Abeywickrama K, Soulillou J. Randomized trial of basiliximab versus placebo for control of acute cellular rejection in renal allograft recipients. *Lancet* 1997;350:1193-1198.

16. Kovarik J, Breidenbach T, Gerbeau C, Korn A, Schmidt AG, Nashan B. Disposition and immunodynamics of basiliximab in liver allograft recipients. *Clin Pharmaco & Therapeu* 1998;64:66-72.

17. Vincenti F, Nashan B, Light S. Daclizumab: Outcome of phase III trials and mechanism of action. *Transplant Proc* 1998;30:2155-2158.

18. Ekberg H, Backman L, Tufveson G, Tyden G. Zenapax (daclizumab) reduces the incidence of acute rejection episodes and improves patient survival following renal transplantation. *Transplant Proc* 1999;31:267-268.

19. Brenner TL, Adams VR. First mAb approved for treatment of metastatic breast cancer. *J Am Pharm Assoc* 1999;39:236-288.

20. Baselga J, Norton L, Albanell J, Kim Y, Mendelsohn J. Recombinant humanized anti-HER2 antibody (herceptin) enhances the antitumor activity of paclitaxel and doxorubicin against HER2/*neu* overexpressing human breast cancer xenografts. *Cancer Res* 1998;58:2825-2831.

21. Pegram MD, Lipton A, Hayes DF, Weber BL, Baselga JM, Tripathy D, Baly D, Baughman SA, Twaddell T, Glaspy JA. Phase II study of receptor-enhanced chemosensitivity using recombinant humanized anti-p185HER2/*neu* monoclonal antibody plus cisplatin in patients with HER2/*neu*-overexpressing metastatic breast cancer refractory to chemotherapy treatment. *J Clin Oncol* 1998;16;2659-2671.

22. Product Information: Herceptin, trastuzumab. Genentech, Inc., San Francisco, CA, 1998.

23. Johnson S, Oliver C, Prince GA, Hemming VG, Pfarr DS, Wang SC, Dormitzer M, O'Grady J, Koenig S, Tamura JK. Development of a humanized monoclonal antibody (MEDI-493) with potent in vitro and in vivo activity against respiratory syncytial virus. *J Infect Dis* 1997;176:1215-1224.

24. Everitt DE, Davis CB, Thompson K, DiCicco R, Ilson B, Demuth SG, Herzyk DJ, Jorkasky DK. The pharmacokinetics, antigenicity, and fusion-inhibition activity of RSHZ19, a humanized monoclonal antibody to respiratory syncytial virus, in healthy volunteers. *J Infect Dis* 1996;174:463-469.

25. Saez-Llorens X, Castano E, Null D, Steichen J, Sanchez PJ, Ramilo O, Top FH Jr., Connor E. Safety and pharmacokinetics of an intramuscular humanized monoclonal antibody to respiratory syncytial virus in premature infants and infants with bronchopulmonary dysplasia. *Ped Infect Dis J* 1998;17:787-791.

26. Product Information: Synagis, Palivizumab. Medimmune, Inc. Rockville, MD, 1999.

27. Anonymous. Palivizumab, a humanized respiratory syncytial virus monoclonal antibody, reduces hospitalizations from respiratory syncytial virus infection in high-risk infants. *Pediatrics* 1998;102:531-537.

Chapter 3

Clotting Factors

Amir Aminimanizani
Parul Patel
Stan G. Louie

INTRODUCTION

The process of coagulation is dependent on a number of factors. Inflammation or trauma to tissues or blood vessels, prosthetic devices, and slowing of blood flow all lead to the formation and activation of various clotting factors. The coagulation cascade starts with either the intrinsic or extrinsic pathway (Figure 3.1). The primary factor responsible for the activation of the intrinsic pathway is factor XII. When factor XII comes into contact with collagen from damaged blood vessels, or attaches to foreign substances, such as prosthetic devices, it initiates the clotting cascade.[1] Factor VIII is also an essential cofactor in modulating the activity of factor IX (FIX) in the intrinsic coagulation pathway.[2]

The extrinsic pathway begins with any sort of vascular damage, which releases a tissue factor, thromboplastin. This tissue factor combines with and activates clotting factor VII, a vitamin K-dependent glycoprotein that plays an important role in the coagulation cascade.[3,4] Factor VII in itself is not active until it forms a complex with tissue factor (TF) at the site of tissue injury to become activated FVII (FVIIa), which can initiate the clotting cascade.[5] From this point on, the intrinsic and extrinsic pathways follow a similar course, leading to the eventual formation of a fibrin clot.[1]

Hemophilia is a group of bleeding disorders that is considered an inherited disease. It can be classified as either Type A (classical hemophilia) or Type B (Christmas disease). Classical hemophilia is a hereditary bleeding disorder characterized by a deficiency of clotting

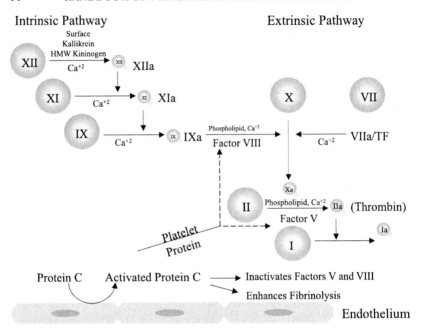

FIGURE 3.1. Coagulation Cascade

factor VIII (FVIII). It is a result of genetic mutations that prevent or reduce the synthesis or the activity of factor VIII.[2]

Alternatively, Type B hemophilia involves a deficiency in factor IX. It is an X-linked hemorrhagic disorder caused by mutations or deletions of the factor IX gene on the long arm of the X-chromosome.[6,7] Factor IX is a vitamin K-dependent clotting factor that binds to the factor VIII-lipid complex, thus activating factor X, which is an essential step in the coagulation cascade.

There are various degrees of hemophilia, classified as severe, moderate, and mild. The degree of severity is determined by the biological activity of the various clotting factors. When the clotting factors have less than 1 percent of normal activity, this is classified as a severe form. Moderate hemophilia occurs when the biological activity is between 1 to 5 percent of normal, whereas mild hemophilia is greater than 5 percent of normal activity.[8]

The frequency of severe to moderate forms of hemophilia is approximately 50 percent. These individuals will require treatment consisting of clotting factor transfusions or cryoprecipitates. The clinical presentation of hemophilia is bleeding from muscles and soft tissues. Internal hemorrhage can also occur from visceral organs, such as severe gastrointestinal bleeding and intra-abdominal hemorrhages. These types of bleeding episodes can usually be managed medically; however, cerebral hemorrhage is a constant risk, which may lead to dire consequences.[8] Essentially, the treatment of hemophilia A involves the replacement of the deficient or inactive FVIII, either for prophylaxis or acute bleeding episodes. The revolutionary development of plasma-derived factor VIII (pd-FVIII) concentrates had led to a new standard in hemophilia care.[9] For almost all cases of hemophilia A, factor concentrates were the treatment and prophylaxis of choice. However, for milder cases, desmopressin (DDAVP) has been proven to be an effective alternative by ensuring hemostasis in mild-to-moderate hemorrhagic events. In fact, doses of 0.3 μg/kg were shown to induce increases in factor VIII:C, von Willebrand factor, and t-PA.[10]

Other than DDAVP, the main treatment options for hemophilia A have been limited by the development of inhibitors to the deficient factor. Also, similar to the transfusion of other blood products, the risk of transmitting bloodborne diseases, such as HIV, hepatitis B, and hepatitis C, are also potential problems associated with the treatment.[2,11,12,13]

Isolated factors from humans can also elicit an immune response, as evident by the formation of neutralizing antibodies or alloantibodies. Neutralizing antibodies are oftentimes referred to as inhibitors. Approximately 20 to 30 percent of individuals with hemophilia A naturally develop inhibitors toward FVIII, and only 1 to 2 percent of patients with hemophilia B developed inhibitors toward FIX.[14] Also, approximately 25 percent of patients given FVIII products develop inhibitors, which deactivates the clotting factors.[15] Although alloantibodies are more likely to develop with longer duration of treatment, most patients develop them before age 20. The development of inhibitors can drastically affect the ability to treat these disorders effectively, thereby seriously compromising patient care.

With respect to hemophilia B, this disorder can be treated by simply replacing sufficient amounts of factor IX to correct the bleeding

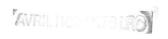

episode.[6,7] The key to treatment is deciding the minimum dose and frequency with which to give factor IX that will achieve proper hemostasis. The amount of factor IX given will vary depending on the clinical presentation at hand. Smaller, less frequent doses are needed for minor hemorrhages and prophylaxis; larger doses are required for surgeries and moderate to severe bleeding episodes.[7]

Traditionally, the only effective therapies for hemophilia B came in the form of intravenously administered plasma-derived factor IX. Fresh, frozen plasma (FFP) was the original source of factor IX for these patients. However, volume restrictions and the high possibility of viral transmission limited the use of this treatment modality.[7] Next, the prothrombin complex concentrates (PCC) consisting of a number of vitamin K-dependent clotting factors, including factor VII, IX, X, proteins C and S, and prothrombin, were developed. The limitations of this formulation include the risk of infectious viral transmission and the possibility of thromboembolic complications such as deep vein thrombosis, pulmonary embolism, and disseminated intravascular coagulation.[7] Highly purified factor IX concentrates were later developed as an attempt to minimize the complications from previous formulations. These concentrates came in two forms, alpha-nine and mononine. Alpha-nine contains only factors IX and X and is purified using the solvent-detergent method. This formulation claims to be virus free and does not predispose patients to thromboembolic complications. Mononine is highly purified factor IX containing no other vitamin K-dependent clotting factors. This formulation is prepared using the monoclonal antibody purification process. Again, the product claims to be free of viruses or thromboembolic complications.[7] Despite these claims, there have been reports of isolated human parvovirus 19 and hepatitis C virus in these products.[5] In addition, these products contain significant amounts of inactive, high molecular weight aggregates of factor IX, which may decrease the specificity of the active clotting factor.[16]

Recent advances in recombinant DNA technology have allowed for the development of several recombinant products that can help treat the various hemophilias, while lowering the risk of transmitting bloodborne pathogens and reducing the development of inhibitors.

RECOMBINANT FACTOR VIIa (NovoSeven®)

Introduction

Recombinant factor VIIa (FVIIa) was developed to provide an alternative therapeutic modality for the treatment of hemorrhagic events in patients with inhibitor development.[14] In vivo, recombinant FVIIa forms a complex with TF at the site of injury, and converts factor X (FX) to activated factor X (FXa), thus leading to hemostasis. This process is independent of factors VIII and IX, is not a systemic reaction, and is not affected by preexisting inhibitors.[5,14,17] Due to these limitations, recombinant coagulation factor IX has also been developed to provide adequate hemostasis without the possibility of viral transmission or thromboembolic complications.

Product Information

Recombinant factor VIIa (rFVIIa) is a recombinant glycoprotein with 406 amino acids and a molecular weight of 50 kDa.[3] An in vitro study found that rFVIIa had identical biological activity as that of plasma-derived factor VIIa.[17] rFVIIa is produced by transfecting baby hamster kidney cells (BHK) with the cDNA containing human FVII gene. The harvested rFVIIa is purified using Mab immunoaffinity and ion exchange chromatography.[5] Subsequently, rFVIIa is autoactivated to yield FVIIa.[5,17]

Viral inactivation is achieved by using the solvent/detergent method that is commonly used for blood-derived products. The final product does not require human or animal albumin for stabilization, further reducing the risk of viral transmission.[17]

rFVIIa has demonstrated a low degree of immunogenicity according to a study of 28 patients treated with multiple doses. No evidence of inhibitor formation was found for up to five months of therapy.[18]

Pharmacokinetics

Pharmacokinetic analysis shows that rFVIIa has an elimination half-life of approximately 2.4 hours with a maximum achieved concentration (Cmax) of 20.0 U/mL after a 70 µg/kg dose.[19] In addition, it appears that plasma FVII:C levels need to be maintained above 6 U/mL to achieve adequate hemostasis.[19]

Clinical Trials

rFVIIa was used on a compassionate basis on 43 patients to treat 51 separate bleeding episodes from 1989 to 1994.[14] Twenty-six (60 percent) patients had hemophilia A with anti-FVIII antibodies, and 30 percent had acquired FVIII inhibitors. All patients were refractory to other therapeutic modalities.[14] These patients received a mean of 80 doses, at an average of 84 µg/kg per dose. An excellent response was observed in 76 percent of the patients with rFVIIa, while only 24 percent showed partially effective or ineffective responses.[14]

rFVIIa was studied in 21 patients with central nervous system (CNS) bleeds.[20] The study investigated the effect of rFVIIa in 16 hemophilia A patients, two with hemophilia B, and three FVII-deficient patients with high inhibitor titers. rFVIIa was used to treat 29 CNS bleeds, with a mean dosage range of 80 to 100 µg/kg ranging from 2 to 332 administrations.[20] Overall efficacy in the hemophilia A patients was reported at 82 percent with one fatality. Similar efficacy (86 percent) was seen with rFVIIa in the hemophilia B and FVII-deficient patients.[20]

The efficacy of rFVIIa was also examined in the treatment of joint and muscle hemorrhagic episodes in 111 hemophilia A and B patients with the presence of inhibitors in the blood.[21] rFVIIa was used in a total of 346 joint and 148 muscle bleeding episodes, which were evaluated 8 and 24 hours after the start of treatment. rFVIIa was administered at a dose ranging from 60 to 120 µg/kg until bleeding was controlled or stopped. The number of doses ranged from 1 to 455, with duration ranging from 2 to 10 days depending on the site and type of bleed.[21] Final evaluation showed that 79 percent of joint bleeds and 69 percent of muscle bleeds were rated as excellent or effective in response to rFVIIa administration. This is compared to only 20 percent of joint bleeds and 29 percent of muscle bleeds that were rated as partially effective in response to FVIIa.[21]

Dosage and Administration

Recombinant factor VIIa has not yet been approved for use in the United States by the FDA.

FACTOR VIII

Introduction

In essence, hemophilia A is an X-linked recessive disorder that affects approximately 1 in 10,000 males. Severe forms of the disease can lead to life-threatening, spontaneous bleeds, in addition to severe hemophilic arthropathy.[11,12]

In healthy individuals, the mature, inactive factor VIII protein has 2,332 amino acids that circulate in the blood as a heterodimer, consisting of domains A1, A2, B, A3, C1, and C2.[5] The factor remains in the bloodstream until needed, and is stabilized by interacting with von Willebrand factor. During activation, factor VIII undergoes proteolytic cleavage, in the process losing the B domain with no apparent loss in activity[5] (Figure 3.2).

cDNA for Factor VIII

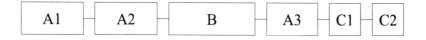

Inactive form of FVIII prior to proteolytic cleavage and activation

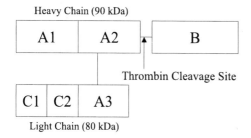

FIGURE 3.2. Factor VIII activation process

ANTIHEMOPHILIC FACTOR (RECOMBINANT)
(Recombinate™)

Product Information

Recombinate or recombinant antihemophilic factor (rAHF) is indicated for the prevention and control of spontaneous hemorrhagic episodes in patients with hemophilia A. It is also indicated as surgical prophylaxis for the patients with hemophilia.[22]

Pharmacology

rAHF is a genetically engineered glycoprotein consisting of a heavy chain and light chain with a molecular weight of 90 to 230 kDa and 70 to 80 kDa, respectively.[23] cDNA encoding for both human factor VIII and von Willebrand factor (vWF) was expressed in chinese hamster ovary (CHO) cells. vWF is added to improve the yield and stability of the crude rAHF.[5,17,22] Since CHO cells require bovine serum albumin for survival, the crude rAHF was purified using murine monoclonal antibody immunoaffinity and ion exchange chromatography techniques.[5,17] The recombinant product was then heated to 40°C for up to eight hours to inactivate enveloped and nonenveloped viruses. Finally, the vWF was removed and human serum albumin was added to stabilize the final product.[5,17] The final rAHF is similar in structure to endogenous FVIII and has an activity of approximately 3,000 IU/mg.[2]

There are no reports of viral transmission directly attributed to the use of rAHF. However, the potential for transmission does exist. There have been reports of human parvovirus B19 DNA isolated from vials of rAHF, which has been attributed to the use of human albumin in the final product.[24]

Besides the fear of viral transmission, the development of inhibitors to factor VIII is also a concern with the introduction of these new recombinant products. Many clinical trials have shown that rAHF can induce low-level inhibitor synthesis. Approximately 31 percent of previously untreated patients have shown inhibitor formation once introduced to rAHF.[5] These inhibitors developed within a few days (mean: 9 to 11 days) after first exposure, and tended to disappear spontaneously thereafter.[5] When compared to patients receiving plasma-derived FVIII concentrates, none of the recombinant factor

VIII products induced the formation of major inhibitors, compared to almost 35 percent of patients receiving pd-FVIII products.[2]

Pharmacokinetics

A pharmacokinetic study comparing rAHF to plasma-derived FVIII products showed that both had similar pharmacokinetic characteristics in a number of categories. Following administration of rAHF, Cmax was determined to be 172.2 IU/dL, while the mean plasma recovery of rAHF was 21.8 IU/dL.[22,25] Serum half-life was 14.5 hours with a clearance 3.1 mL/kg per hour. Volume of distribution was estimated to be 61.9 mL/kg.[25]

Clinical Trials

In a prospective, open-label, multicenter trial, 69 previously treated patients with moderate to severe hemophilia A were assigned to receive either Recombinate or plasma-derived FVIII to assess the efficacy and safety of the recombinant product. Patients were assigned to receive Recombinate for prophylaxis and treatment of all bleeding episodes for a period of 1 to 5.7 years.[23] During the study, a total of 17,700 infusions of rAHF were administered, with an average dose of 27.5 IU/kg per patient, and mean of 241 exposure days per patient. A total of 6,440 episodes of bleeding were treated, with 91.2 percent of the episodes determined to have a treatment rating of excellent to good. The percentage of episodes with a fair rating was 7.2 percent, and < 1 percent (0.89 percent) were rated as no response.[23] Thirteen of these patients were given rAHF for surgical prophylaxis in 24 separate procedures. All 24 procedures were given a rating of excellent, without any unexpected incidents or excessive blood loss.[23]

A prospective, open-labeled trial evaluating the safety and efficacy of rAHF was conducted in 73 severe hemophilia A patients who were treatment naive.[26] All patients were treated either in response to an acute hemorrhagic episode or as procedural prophylaxis. A total of 1,785 infusions were administered to treat 810 hemorrhagic episodes for an average of 11 treatment days. Results showed that 92 percent of all episodes responded well to one or two rAHF infusions. There were also 10 invasive procedures, ranging from central venous catheter placement to lumbar puncture that were treated with recombinant factor VIII. In 9 of 10 procedures, the quality of hemostasis achieved was rated as excellent.[26]

Adverse Reactions

During various clinical trials, 13 infusion-related adverse reactions were reported from 13,394 infusions (0.097 percent).[22,23] Reactions included slight flushing, nausea, sneezing, and brief dizziness shortly after the infusion.[23] In one trial, erythematous rash was reported during 2 of 1,785 (0.1 percent) infusions.[26]

Dosage and Administration

Dosing of rAHF will depend on the level of antihemophilic factor (AHF) required to achieve hemostasis. The expected AHF increase, expressed as IU/dL or percent of normal, can be estimated by multiplying the dose (IU/kg) by two.[22] For example, a dose of 25 IU/kg can be expected to raise AHF levels to 50 percent of normal (25 IU/kg × 2). Duration of treatment will depend on desired level of hemostasis and clinical situation (Table 3.1).

Preparation and Storage

rAHF is supplied as a sterile, lyophilized powder that is available in single-dose vials of 250, 500, or 1000 IU per bottle.[22] rAHF should not be frozen, but stored at 2° to 8°C (36° to 46°F) or at room temperature not to exceed 30°C (86°F). The reconstituted rAHF should be administered within three hours after admixtured.[22]

ANTIHEMOPHILIC FACTOR (RECOMBINANT)
(Kogenate®)

Product Information

Kogenate is indicated for the treatment of hemophilia A, in which there is evidence of deficiency in the activity of clotting factor VIII.[27]

TABLE 3.1. Dosing Guidelines for Recombinate

Degree of Hemorrhage	Required Postinfusion AHF Activity (% of normal or IU/dL)	Frequency
Early hemarthrosis, muscle bleed, oral bleed	20-40	Administer every 12-24 hours for 1-3 days, or until bleeding has resolved or healing is achieved
More extensive hemarthrosis, muscle bleed, hematoma	30-60	Repeat infusion every 12-24 hours for 3 days or until pain/disability is resolved
Life-threatening bleeds, such as head injury, throat bleeds, severe abdominal pain	60-100	Repeat infusion every 8-24 hours until bleeding has resolved
Minor surgery, including tooth extraction	60-80	Single infusion plus oral antifibrinolytic therapy within 1 hour of procedure
Major surgery	80-100 (pre- and postop)	Repeat every 8-24 hours depending on the amount of healing

Source: Product Information: Recombinate™, Recombinant Antihemophilic Factor VIII. Baxter Healthcare, Glendale, CA, 1998.

Pharmacology

Kogenate is an engineered glycoprotein consisting of a heavy and light chain, weighing 90 and 80 kDa, respectively. Kogenate is produced by transfecting baby hamster kidney (BHK) cells with the cDNA for human factor VIII genes.[5,17,28]

Similar to other mammalian expression systems, BHK cells are cultured in a medium containing bovine serum-free medium, allowing for high recovery of rFVIII without the need for von Willebrand factor to stabilize the protein.[5,17] The raw rAHF is processed through a multistep purification process, including monoclonal murine antibody immunoaffinity.[29] The product is then heat treated at 40°C for eight hours to inactivate viral contaminants. Human serum albumin is then added to stabilize the final product.[5]

Similar to other rAHF, no reports of viral transmission have been attributed to Kogenate. In fact, two studies have shown that no study patient had seroconverted for a specific virus as a result of receiving Kogenate.[11,28] However, in one study, 5 of 16 susceptible patients seroconverted for parvovirus B19 after therapy.[13] After intensive analysis, investigators could not rule out the possibility of parvovirus B19 transmission from Kogenate in two of the five patients.[13] As with Recombinate, the source of the virus is believed to be the human albumin used as a stabilizer in the final formulation.

Inhibitor development is the second concern regarding the use of recombinant antihemophilic factors. In one study, 16 of 81 patients (20 percent) developed inhibitors to factor VIII after treatment with Kogenate.[28] Inhibitor titers were low in 9 of the 16 patients despite continuous treatment with Kogenate. The inhibitors completely disappeared in 4 of 16 patients, and remained low in 5 of 16 patients.[28] In another study, inhibitors developed in 8 of 107 patients (7.5 percent) treated with Kogenate.[11] As in the previous study, inhibitor titers remained low despite continuous treatment. In another clinical trial, there was no evidence of inhibitor formation in 39 patients treated with Kogenate.[13]

Pharmacokinetics

Kogenate has pharmacokinetic characteristics similar to plasma-derived factor VIII formulations. One study demonstrated Kogenate as having an elimination half-life of approximately 15.76 hours and the estimated clearance of 2.49 mL/kg per hour. The volume of distribution was determined to be 50.54 mL/kg.[11]

Clinical Trials

An open-label, multicenter trial examined the safety and efficacy of Kogenate in 39 previously treated patients with hemophilia A. Recombinant FVIII was administered for prophylaxis and treatment of bleeding episodes, with patients or physicians subjectively assessing the efficacy of the product.[13] At the end of the trial, 3,679 infusions were administered with a median of 68.5 exposure days per patient. Of the 3,679 infusions, 1,439 were assessed for efficacy in treating bleeding episodes. The treatment was considered to be successful or very successful for 1,292 of the 1,439 infusions (89.8 percent).[13]

Only 147 infusions (10.2 percent) were considered fair or not successful. Of 844 bleeding episodes examined, 759 (89.9 percent) were treated with one or two infusions.[13]

Another open-label, multicenter study analyzed the safety and efficacy of Kogenate in 26 patients with hemophilia A. The patients were treated for surgical procedures or serious hemorrhages requiring hospitalization.[11] The 26 patients were treated for 22 separate major surgical procedures such as joint replacements, dental surgery, laparotomy, and orthopedic surgery. There were also ten occasions of in-hospital serious hemorrhages. On all 32 occasions, hemostasis was rated as excellent.[11]

Adverse Reactions

During clinical trials, only 47 of 12,932 infusions (0.36 percent) were associated with minor adverse events.[27] The reactions reported were primarily infusion related such as flushing, headache, pain at injection site, pruritis, dizziness, rash, and erythema.[11,13,27]

Dosage and Administration

Similar to Recombinate, the dosage of Kogenate is dependent on the clinical situation. The severity of FVIII deficiency, severity of hemorrhage, the presence of inhibitors, and the level of AHF will determine the dosage of Kogenate required (Table 3.2). The dose required is calculated using the equation below:[27]

$$\text{Dose Required (IU)} = \frac{\text{Body Weight (kg)} \times \text{Desired \% Factor Increase}}{2 \text{ \%/IU/kg}}$$

Preparation and Storage

Kogenate is supplied as a sterile, lyophilized powder for injection, which is available in single-dose vials of 250, 500, and 1,000 IU per bottle.[27] Kogenate is to be stored at 2° to 8°C (36° to 46°F). At room temperature (25°C), the product may be stored for as long as three months. This product should not be stored in freezing conditions. As with other clotting factors, Kogenate solution should be administered within three hours after reconstitution.[27]

TABLE 3.2. Dosage Guidelines for Kogenate

Degree of Hemorrhage	Required Postinfusion AHF Activity (% of normal or IU/dL)	Frequency
Mild hemorrhage	20	One dose, unless further doses are required
Moderate hemorrhage	30-50	Repeat infusions every 12-24 hours until resolved
Severe hemorrhage	80-100	Repeat every 8-12 hours until bleeding has resolved
Surgery	100	Preoperative dose, then repeat infusions every 6-12 hours as needed for 10-14 days, or until healing is complete

Source: Product Information: Kogenate®, Recombinant Antihemophilic Factor VIII. Bayer Corporation, Elkhart, IN, 2001.

RECOMBINANT, B-DOMAIN DELETED FACTOR VIII, r-FVIII SQ (Refacto®)

Product Information

Refacto is currently under investigation for approval for the treatment of hemorrhagic episodes in patients with hemophilia A. This product is an rFVIII fragment with molecular weight of 170 kDa which is missing the central B-domain.[9]

Pharmacology

This product has two heavy and light chains with molecular weights of 90 kDa and 80 kDa, respectively.[9,17] Similar to other recombinant clotting factors, FVIII SQ is produced by transfecting cDNA encoding for human FVIII which is lacking the B-domain into CHO cells.[5] The crude rFVIII SQ is purified through a number of chromatographic methods that begin with ion exchange, size exclusion, and finally immunoaffinity chromatography.

Viral inactivation is accomplished using the solvent/detergent method.[5] No human albumin or von Willebrand factor is added to the final product, as stabilization with these products is not necessary. Refacto has been shown to have a specific activity of approximately 15,000 IU/mg, compared to 4,000 to 7,000 IU/mg for the other recombinant FVIII products.[9,12]

A trial conducted on 36 patients with hemophilia A found no incidents of viral transmission. This may be expected in this product since the final preparation does not contain any human or animal proteins, as is required for the other recombinant factor VIII products. No new inhibitors were found to factor VIII during the trial and up to two weeks after the last infusion.[12] In another trial, 10 of 72 (14 percent) patients treated with Refacto developed inhibitors within a mean of 9.5 days after the start of therapy.[30]

Pharmacokinetics

After a 50 IU/kg infusion of Refacto, the Cmax was found to be 1.3 IU/mL.[12] The elimination half-life was determined to be approximately 13 hours, with a clearance of 2.8 mL/kg per hour. The volume of distribution of 45 mL/kg was similar to other clotting factors.

Clinical Trials

In a safety and efficacy trial of 87 hemophilia A patients, Refacto was used to treat various hemorrhagic episodes or for surgical prophylaxis.[30] During the trial, 778 joint bleeds were treated with a mean dose of 30 IU/kg. The response rate was 94 percent after three or fewer injections. The efficacy was rated as excellent in 87 percent of the cases.[30]

During this trial, Refacto was also studied in 17 patients undergoing 22 separate surgical procedures. Hemostasis was rated as excellent in all cases with blood loss equal to that of nonhemophiliacs undergoing similar procedures.[30]

Adverse Reactions

In two separate trials with Refacto, adverse events related to use were extremely rare. In one study there was no incident of adverse reactions during the treatment and up to two weeks after therapy.[12] In another study, there were no adverse reactions associated with the use of Refacto.[30]

Dosage and Administration

Since this product is not yet approved for use in the United States, dosing guidelines are not available. However, as with other recombinant clotting factor products, dosing will depend on the clinical situation and level of inhibition required.

FACTOR IX, rFIX (Benefix®)

Product Information

Recombinant factor IX (rFIX) is indicated for the control and prevention of hemorrhagic episodes in patients with hemophilia B.[31] It is a 550 kDa glycoprotein consisting of 415 amino acids in a single chain, identical to the allelic form of plasma-derived factor IX.[31,32] rFIX has an identical mechanism of action as the native factor IX.

Pharmacology

The product is isolated from CHO cells carrying the cDNA of human FIX.[16,31] rFIX is then secreted into a culture medium that does not contain any proteins derived from human or animal sources, further ensuring the lack of viral transmission.[5,16]

The recombinant formulation technology and a multilayered viral filtration system ensure that rFIX carries no inherent risk of passing on viral pathogens such as HIV, parvovirus, or the family of hepatitis viruses.[31,33] In addition to its viral safety profile, rFIX is also higher in purity and specificity than the previous factor IX formulations. rFIX has less than 1 percent of the high molecular weight inactivated aggregates that can reduce specificity and purity. This is compared to the highly purified factor IX concentrates that contain anywhere from 10 to 50 percent of these aggregates.[16] As a result, rFIX has a specific activity of approximately 270 IU/mg, compared to the highly purified products with specific activities of approximately 90 to 230 IU/mg.[32]

Pharmacokinetics

rFIX has a terminal half-life of approximately 20 hours, which is not significantly different from that of plasma-derived factor IX. For each IU/kg infused, the mean circulating factor IX activity was increased by 0.8 IU/dL.[16,31] In vivo recovery of rFIX was found to be 28 percent lower than in patients receiving plasma-derived factor IX.[16] Similar results were found in studies done on canine models receiving multiple doses of rFIX.[6]

Clinical Trials

An open-label, multicenter study evaluated the safety and efficacy of rFIX in 56 patients with moderate to severe hemophilia B in the management of acute bleeding and surgical prophylaxis.[34,35] All study patients had previously been exposed to plasma-derived factor IX. They were scheduled to receive rFIX as needed for hemorrhagic episodes or for prophylaxis prior to and after surgery. To date, 1,070 hemorrhages occurred, requiring 1,514 transfusions with dosing varying from 6.5 to 125.5 IU/kg.[34,35] Of these 1,070 incidents, up to 80 percent of them were stopped after only one dose of rFIX. In addition, 87 percent of the infusions were rated as providing either similar or superior clinical responses when compared to previous treatment with plasma-derived concentrates.[35]

In another trial, the efficacy of rFIX was examined in 12 patients with hemophilia B undergoing a total of 13 surgical procedures.[36] The surgeries included six orthopedic procedures, four dental extractions, one liver transplant, one hernia repair, and one biopsy of a skin lesion. Dosing of rFIX ranged from 10,000 to 348,000 IU. The results indicated that over 97 percent of cases were rated as excellent in terms of clinical response, with blood loss similar to nonhemophiliacs undergoing the same types of procedures.[36]

Adverse Reactions

In clinical trials, the most commonly reported adverse reaction was nausea, pain at injection site, and altered taste.[31,35] One patient with > 250 exposure days to plasma-derived factor IX and > 39 exposure days to rFIX had reported to develop activity-neutralizing antibodies to factor IX.[35] To date, there have been no reports of viral seroconversion attributed to the use of rFIX. The manufacturer also suggests using rFIX with caution in patients with disseminated intravascular coagulation or other clotting disorders due to the history of thromboembolic complications when other factor IX concentrates are used.[31]

Dosage and Administration

Dosing of rFIX will depend on the severity of factor IX deficiency and clinical presentation. A formula to guide empiric dosing follows.[31]

Units of rFIX required = body wt (kg) × desired factor IX increase (%) × 1.2 IU/kg

Duration of therapy can range from one to ten days depending on the treatment goal (Table 3.3). rFIX is administered by intravenous infusion over several minutes.

Preparation and Storage

Benefix is supplied as a sterile powder for injection in vials containing 250, 500, or 1000 IU of rFIX. The powder should not be frozen, but stored between 2° to 8°C (36° to 46°F). The drug may also be stored at room temperature not exceeding 25°C (77°F) for up to six months. Since the product does not contain any preservatives, it is recommended that reconstituted rFIX be used within three hours.[31]

NOTES

1. Haines ST, Racine E, Zeolla M. Venous thromboembolism. In Dipiro JT, Talbert RL, Yee GC, Matzke GR, Wells BG, Posey LM. (Eds.), *Pharmacotherapy: A pathophysiologic approach,* Third edition, Stamford, CT: Appleton & Lang, 2002, pp. 337-374.

2. Prescott R, Nakai H, Saenko EL, Scharrer I, Nilsson IM, Humphries JE, Hurst D, Bray G, Scandella D. The inhibitor antibody response is more complex in hemophilia A patients than in most nonhemophiliacs with factor VIII auto-antibodies. *Blood* 1997;89(10):3663-3671.

3. Bauer KA. Treatment of factor VII deficiency with recombinant factor VIIa. *Haemostasis* 1996;26(Suppl 1):155-158.

TABLE 3.3. Dosing Guidelines for rFIX

Type of Hemorrhage	Circulating Factor IX Activity Required (%)	Frequency of Doses (h)	Duration (d)
Minor, uncomplicated hemarthroses, superficial muscle, or soft tissue	20-30	12-24	1-2
Moderate intramuscular or soft tissue with dissection, mucous membranes, dental extractions, or hematuria	25-50	12-24	Treat until bleeding stops and healing begins; about 2-7 days
Major pharynx, retropharynx, retroperitoneum, CNS, surgery	50-100	12-24	7-10

Source: Product Information: Benefix®, Recombinant Factor IX. Genetics Institute, Cambridge, MA, 1998.

4. Kristensen J, Killander A, Hippe E, Helleberg C, Ellegard J, Holm M, Kutti J, Mellqvist UH, Johansson JE, Glazer S. Clinical experience with recombinant factor VIIa in patients with thrombocytopenia. *Haemostasis* 1996;26 (Suppl 1):159-164.

5. Roddie PH, Ludlam CA. Recombinant coagulation factors. *Haemostasis and Thrombosis* 1997;11:169-177.

6. Brinkhous KM, Sigman JL, Read MS, Stewart PF, McCarthy KP, Timony GA, Leppanen SD, Rup BJ, Keith JC Jr., Garzone PD. Recombinant human factor IX: Replacement therapy, orophylaxis, and pharmacokinetics in canine hemophilia B. *Blood* 1996;88(7):2603-2610.

7. Roberts HR, Eberst ME. Current management of hemophilia B. *Hematology/Oncology Clinics of North America* 1993;7(3):1269-1280.

8. Fauci AS, Harrison TR, et al. (Eds.), *Harrison's principles of internal medicine,* Fourteenth edition. New York: McGraw-Hill, Health Professions Division, 1998.

9. Berntorp E. The treatment of haemophilia, including prophylaxis, constant infusion and DDAVP. *Balliere's Clinical Haematology* 1996;9(2):259-271.

10. Mannucci PM, Canciani MT, Rota L, Donovan RD. Response of factor VIII/von Willebrand factor to DDAVP in healthy subjects, and patients with hemophilia A, and von Willebrand's disease. *British Journal of Haemotology* 1981; 47:283-293.

11. Schwartz RS, Abildgaard CF, Aledort LM, Arkin S, Bloom AL, Brackmann HH, Brettler DB, Fukui H, Hilgartner MW, Inwood MJ. Human recombinant DNA-

derived antihemophilic factor (factor VIII) in the treatment of hemophilia A. *New England Journal of Medicine* 1990;323(26):1800-1805.

12. Fijnvandraat K, Berntorp E, ten Cate JW, Johnsson H, Peters M, Savidge G, Tengborn L, Spira J, Stahl C. Recombinant, B-domain deleted factor VIII (r-VII SQ): Pharmacokinetics and initial safety aspects in hemophilia A patients. *Thrombosis and Haemostasis* 1997;77(2):298-302.

13. Aygoren-Pursun E, Scharrer I. A multicenter pharmacosurveillance study for the evaluation of the efficacy and safety of recombinant factor VIII in the treatment of patients with hemophilia A. *Thrombosis and Haemostasis* 1997;78:1352-1356.

14. Lusher JM. Recombinant factor VIIa (NovoSeven) in the treatment of internal bleeding in patients with factor VIII and IX inhibitors. *Haemostasis* 1996;26 (Suppl 1):124-130.

15. Hoyer LW, Scandella D. Factor VIII inhibitors: Structure and function in autoantibody and hemophilia A patients. *Seminars in Hematology* 1994;31:1.

16. White GC, Beebe A, Nielsen B. Recombinant factor IX. *Thrombosis and Haemostasis* 1997;78(1):261-265.

17. Lusher JM. Recombinant clotting factor concentrates. *Balliere's Clinical Haematology* 1996;9(2):291-303.

18. Nicolaisen EM. Long-term follow-up with regard to potential immunogenicity: Clinical experience with NovoSeven. *Haemostasis* 1996;26 (Suppl 1):98-101.

19. Hedner U. Dosing and monitoring of NovoSeven treatment. *Haemostasis* 1996;26 (Suppl 1):102-108.

20. Rice KM, Savidge GF. NovoSeven (recombinant factor VIIa) in central nervous system bleeds. *Haemostasis* 1996;26 (Suppl 1):131-134.

21. Bech RM. Recombinant factor VIIa in joint and muscle bleeding episodes. *Haemostasis* 1996;26 (Suppl 1):135-138.

22. Product Information: Recombinate, Recombinant Antihemophilic Factor VIII. Baxter Healthcare, Glendale, CA, 1998.

23. White GC, Courter S, Bray GL, Lee M, Gomperts ED. A multicenter study of recombinant factor VIII (Recombinate) in previously treated patients with hemophilia A. *Thrombosis and Hemostasis* 1997;77(4):660-667.

24. Eis-Hubinger AM, Sasowski U, Brackmann HH, Kaiser R, Matz B, Schneweis KE. Parvovirus B19 DNA is frequently present in recombinant coagulation factor VIII products. *Thrombosis and Haemostasis* 1996;76:1120.

25. Morfini M, Longo G, Messori A, Lee M, White G, Mannucci P. Pharmacokinetic properties of recombinant factor VIII compared with a monoclonally purified concentrate. *Thrombosis and Hemostasis* 1992;68(4):433-435.

26. Bray GL, Gomperts ED, Courter S, Gruppo R, Gordon EM, Manco-Johnson M, Shapiro A, Scheibel F, White G, Lee M. A multicenter study of recombinant factor VIII (Recombinate): Safety, efficacy, and inhibitor risk in previously untreated patients with hemophilia A. *Blood* 1994;83(9):2428-2435.

27. Product Information: Kogenate, Recombinant Antihemophilic Factor VIII. Bayer Corporation. Elkhart, IN, 2001.

28. Lusher JM, Arkin S, Abildgaard CF, Schwartz RS. Recombinant factor VIII for the treatment of previously untreated patients with hemophilia A-Safety, efficacy, and development of inhibitors. *The New England Journal of Medicine* 1993;328(7):453-459.

29. Lusher JM. Summary of clinical experience with recombinant factor VIII products—Kogenate. *Annals of Haematology* 1994;68 (Suppl S):3-6.

30. Berntorp E. Second generation, B-domain deleted recombinant factor VIII. *Thrombosis and Haemostasis* 1997;78(1):256-260.

31. Product Information: Benefix, Recombinant Factor IX: Genetics Institute, Cambridge, MA, 1998.

32. Bond M, Jankowski M, Patel H, Karnik S, Strang A, Xu B, Rouse J, Koza S, Letwin B, Steckert J. Biochemical characterization of recombinant factor IX. *Seminars in Hematology* 1998;35(2) (Suppl 2):11-17.

33. Adamson S, Charlebois T, O'Connel B, Foster W. Viral safety of recombinant factor IX. *Seminars in Hematology* 1998;35(2) (Suppl 2):22-27.

34. White G, Shapiro A, Lusher J, Roth D, Pasi J, Kentzer T, Courter S. Recombinant factor IX in the treatment of hemorrhage in previously treated patients with hemophilia B. *British Journal of Haemotology* 1996;93 (Suppl 2):163.

35. White G, Shapiro A, Ragni M, Garzone P, Goodfellow J, Tubridy K, Courter S. Clinical evaluation of recombinant factor IX. *Seminars in Hematology* 1998; 35(2) (Suppl 2):33-38.

36. Ragni M, Shapiro A, White G, Pasi J, Laurian Y, Gencavella N, Quiles E, Courier S. Use of recombinant factor IX in six patients with hemophilia B undergoing surgery. *British Journal of Haematology* 1996;93 (Suppl 2):163.

Chapter 4

Enzymes and Regulators
of Enzymatic Activity

Jay P. Rho
Jennifer Cupo-Abbott
Stan G. Louie
Parul Patel

INTRODUCTION

Several attributes of enzymes make them especially suitable as drugs, including their reaction specificity, their catalytic efficiency, and their capacity to operate under mild conditions of temperature alterations. In cancer chemotherapy, L-asparaginase has long been a useful adjunct in the treatment of acute lymphoblastic leukemia, but recent experience suggests a role in acute nonlymphoblastic leukemia as well. The replacement of genetically deficient enzymes in patients with inherited metabolic disorders by infusion of purified enzymes or by organ transplantation has had very limited success, although good results with bone marrow transplantation have been obtained in some patients with cystic fibrosis, Gaucher's disease, and inherited immunodeficiency diseases. Treatment of chronic pancreatic insufficiency and of disaccharidase deficiency with oral enzymes can be very effective; therapy can be monitored in the latter by measuring the breath hydrogen excretion and in the former by a range of tests, of which stool chymotrypsin assay is the most convenient. Treatment of acute myocardial infarction by intracoronary perfusion of thrombolytic enzymes can improve both cardiac function and long-term survival if administered early enough. Successful reperfusion can be identified by changes in the kinetics of serum enzyme release and clearance, especially for the isoenzymes and isoforms of creatine kinase. Controlled enzymatic activation and fibrinolysis with alteplase, reteplase, lanoteplase, and tenecteplase are important therapeutic advances in the management of thromboembolic vascular disease.

Microorganisms have generally been the source of therapeutic enzymes. Large quantities of a microorganism can be cultured at relatively low cost and in a short time frame. Recombinant technology has been a major therapeutic advance in improving the specificity of enzyme production and in lowering the immunogenicity of purified enzymes.

ALTEPLASE (Activase®)

Acute coronary syndromes may clinically manifest as unstable angina and acute myocardial infarction (AMI). Under normal physiologic conditions, circulating blood components do not normally interact with intact vascular endothelium. However, circulating blood components will interact with disrupted or dysfunctional surfaces. A series of biochemical events will give rise to the rapid deposition of blood cells and the formation of insoluble fibrin. Thrombus forming in the arterial system is usually composed of platelets and fibrin. In contrast, venous thrombi usually consist of erythrocytes and fibrin, where aggregated platelets are also present.

A critical step in arterial thrombosis formation is platelet attachment onto nonendothelial or disrupted surfaces. This is followed by adherence, activation, and aggregation along the involved area, where a rapid enlargement of platelet mass begins to form. Under physiologic conditions, this represents a primary step in hemostasis. In pathologic thrombosis, platelet adherence initiates a process that, if poorly regulated, can ultimately lead to vessel occlusion.

Thrombin formation in coronary arteries may impair coronary artery flow, thus becomes the impetus of acute myocardial infarction. Rapid dissolution of the clot may preserve myocardial tissues, thus preventing ischemia and tissue necrosis. Prolonged ischemia or tissue necrosis can lead to heart failure and increased risk of death. Natural fibrinolysis is mediated by plasmin, the active form of plasminogen. Tissue plasminogen activators mediate the activation of plasmin, which may be used to dissolve clots.

Product Information

Alteplase is recombinant human tissue plasminogen activator (tPA) produced by inserting complementary DNA encoding for tPA expressed in CHO (chinese hamster ovary) cells.[1] The resultant glycoprotein has a polypeptide backbone consisting of 527 amino acids. Structurally, alteplase is a 78 kD serine protease containing three carbohydrate side chains and 17 disulfide bonds.

Pharmacology

Alteplase is a serine protease produced through recombinant technology that promotes the conversion of plasminogen to plasmin in the presence of fibrin. However, in the absence of fibrin, tPA causes limited conversion of plasminogen, unlike streptokinase or urokinase.[2]

Systemically, alteplase binds onto fibrin in a thrombus and converts the trapped plasminogen to plasmin, initiating local fibrinolysis with limited systemic proteolysis. Typically, a 16 to 36 percent decrease in circulating fibrinogen can be expected following a 100 mg dose of alteplase.[3]

Pharmacokinetics

The pharmacokinetic profile of alteplase is based on limited studies conducted in AMI and thrombo-occlusive diseased patients. The mean initial plasma half-life is less than five minutes and the terminal half-life is approximately 30 to 45 minutes.[2] Approximately 80 percent of alteplase is removed from the circulation within ten minutes after discontinuing IV therapy. The plasma clearance of alteplase is 380 to 570 mL/min, which requires dose adjustment in hepatic insufficiency. The initial volume of distribution is approximately that of total plasma volume.[1]

Clinical Trials

Alteplase is approved for use in the management of AMI and acute massive pulmonary embolism in adults. Although not FDA approved, alteplase has also been investigated for use in the treatment of unstable angina pectoris, subarachnoid hemorrhage, superior vena cava thrombosis, and thromboembolic stroke with some success.

An estimated 1.5 million people suffer an AMI each year with an extremely high morbidity and mortality, resulting in one-fourth of all deaths in the United States.[1] Several studies have demonstrated the benefits of early administration of thrombolytic agents. These benefits include an improvement in ventricular function, a lower incidence of cardiogenic shock, and a reduction in overall mortality. Thrombolytic therapy involves enzymatic dissolution of a thrombus by breaking down the fibrin network. As mentioned previously, alteplase binds to fibrin in a thrombus and converts trapped plasminogen to plasmin, which is the active enzyme. In the absence of fibrin, alteplase has limited abilities to initiate this conversion.

Alteplase is distinct from the four commercially available thrombolytic agents in two areas: (1) alteplase is considered to be clot specific with conversion of plasminogen to plasmin at the clot site and not within the systemic circulation, and (2) alteplase has the highest early infarct artery patency rate (i.e., within 90 minutes of treatment).[1] Despite these differences, considerable debate remains regarding the role of alteplase in clinical practice. Numerous clinical trials have been conducted to elucidate its role.

The GISSI-2 trial and the International Study Group are two multicenter trials that compared the in-hospital mortality for patients treated with streptokinase (a serine protease that is derived from streptococcus) or alteplase within six hours of AMI.[4] No statistical differences in the incidence of combined end point of death or severe left ventricular damage were noted between alteplase and streptokinase, either with or without heparin.[1] Likewise, no significant difference between the two thrombolytic agents was found in patients for the following covariates: time to treatment, age, sex, previous history of MI, and infarct site. The ISIS-3 trial compared the effects of alteplase, streptokinase, and anistreplase on 35-day and six-month mortality in patients admitted within 24 hours of symptom onset.[1] Again, no statistical differences were found among the thrombolytics.

The GUSTO (Global Utilization of Streptokinase and tPA of Occluded Arteries) trial was designed to investigate the benefits of a "front loaded" dose of alteplase (a large initial bolus followed by an infusion of the total dose over 90 minutes) compared with conventional alteplase administration. Safety and improvement in mortality of combining alteplase and streptokinase with either agent alone was also studied. Results from this study appear to show a favorable mortality rate in patients treated with alteplase compared to the streptokinase-treated patients.[1]

Alteplase has also been shown to be effective when used to treat pulmonary embolisms. In one study involving 36 patients with angiographically documented pulmonary embolism, alteplase was shown to induce clot lysis in 34 patients, indicating the efficacy of alteplase for the treatment of pulmonary embolism.[1] Alteplase was administered at a dose of 50 mg over two hours followed by an additional 40 mg over four hours if clot lysis had not occurred.

Although there are no well-controlled studies examining the use of alteplase in the treatment of subarachnoid hemorrhages, a number of case reports suggest alteplase may be effective in the prevention of vasospasm and delayed ischemia secondary to subarachnoid hemorrhage.[1] Alteplase was given as a single intracisternal bolus intraoperatively or as multiple intrathecal doses postoperative. Bleeding complications remain the primary concern. One investigator reported the use of alteplase in the treatment of basilar artery occlusion, where recannulization of the entire basilar artery was observed at 90 minutes and 20 hours after the initiation of fibrinolysis by angiographic methods.[1] Other reports include the use of alteplase in patients with an intra-arterial infusion and an acute cerebral arterial occlusion.[1]

Adverse Reactions

Bleeding is the most frequently observed adverse effect associated with alteplase. Bleeding can be internal, involving the gastrointestinal tract, genitourinary tract, retroperitoneal or intracranial sites, or the bleeding can be superficial, observed mainly at invaded or disturbed sites such as venous cutdowns and arterial puncture sites.[1] Concomitant use of anticoagulants, such as heparin, can increase the risk of bleeding. If serious bleeding is detected, alteplase infusion should be immediately stopped and supportive care should be initiated. Other adverse reactions noted include occasional mild hypersensitivity reactions. Nausea, vomiting, hypotension, and fever often occur, but may be due to sequelae of acute myocardial infarction and not the drug itself.[1]

Dosage and Administration

The dosage of alteplase is dependent on body weight (not to exceed 100 mg), the indication, and the type of infusion. In AMI patients receiving an accelerated infusion with a weight equal to or greater than 67 kg , the recommended dosage is 100 mg administered as a 15 mg IV bolus, followed by 50 mg infused over 30 minutes, and then 35 mg infused over the next 60 minutes.[2] AMI patients undergoing a three-hour infusion with the aforementioned weight profile should be given 100 mg of alteplase administered 60 mg in the first hour (of which 6 to 10 mg is administered as a bolus), 20 mg over the second hour, and 20 mg over the third hour.[1]

The alteplase dose for the treatment of adult patients with acute pulmonary embolism is 100 mg by IV infusion administered over two hours with heparin as recommended.[2] For the treatment of acute ischemic stroke, the recommended adult dose is 0.9 mg/kg administered over 60 minutes, with 10 percent of the total dose given as an initial IV loading dose over one minute. Alteplase therapy should begin within three hours after stroke and should not exceed the maximum recommended dose of 90 mg. Studies indicate that this regimen of rt-PA was beneficial in reducing disability at three months compared to placebo.[3]

Alteplase is available as a sterile, lyophilized powder in either 50 mg or 100 mg per vial, 29 million IU and 58 million IU, respectively. The product should be used intravenously within eight hours after reconstitution and stored away from excessive light at room temperature under refrigeration (2° to 8°C).[1]

RETEPLASE (Retavase®)

Product Information

Reteplase is a tissue plasminogen activator (tPA) analog that was produced using recombinant technology. It is indicated for the management of acute myocardial infarction (AMI) in adults for ventricular function improvement following AMI and a reduction of congestive heart failure incidence and mortality associated with AMI. Treatment should be initiated as soon as possible after the onset of

AMI symptoms.[5] Comparative FDA-approved indications for the thrombolytic agents are summarized in Table 4.1.[5,6]

Reteplase is a nonglycosylated deletion mutant of wild-type tissue plasminogen activator. It is produced in *Escherichia coli* using recombinant DNA technology. It consists of the kringle-2 and serine protease domains, but lacks the kringle-1, finger, and growth factor domains of tissue plasminogen activator. It is a 355-amino acid polypeptide with a molecular weight of 39 kD.[5]

Reteplase is available in vials containing 10.8 units as a lyophilized powder for intravenous bolus injection after reconstitution. It is packaged in kits containing all the materials necessary for reconstitution. The kits should be stored at 2° to 25°C (36° to 77°F) and protected from light until use.[5]

Pharmacology

Compared to alteplase, reteplase has a longer half-life and greater thrombolytic potency, but weaker affinity for fibrin. However, similar to alteplase, it activates plasminogen directly and does not require plasminogen complexing. Reteplase causes more fibrinogen depletion than alteplase, which could result in a higher frequency of bleeding complications. Yet clinical trials have not demonstrated a difference at this time.[7,8,9] Reteplase is not antigenic and can be administered repeatedly, although there is no report with patients receiving repeated courses of therapy.[5,9]

TABLE 4.1. Comparative FDA-Approved Indications

Indication	Alteplase	Reteplase	Streptokinase
Acute myocardial infarction	X	X	X
Pulmonary embolism	X		X
Deep vein thrombosis			X
Arterial thrombosis or embolism			X
Occlusion of arteriovenous cannulae			X

Source: Product Information: Alteplase. Genentech, Inc., San Francisco, 1999.

Pharmacokinetics

Reteplase is cleared from plasma at a rate of 250 to 450 mL/min. The distribution half-life, which represents the effective half-life of reteplase, is 13 to 16 minutes. Clearance is hepatic and renal.[5] Alteplase, in comparison, has a half-life of less than five minutes. The longer half-life of reteplase allows for bolus dosing of this agent.[6,10]

Clinical Trials

Small studies have been performed to compare patency rates. These studies have demonstrated that reteplase has an effect on survival and is equivalent to that of streptokinase.[9,10,11] Double-bolus administration of reteplase is currently being compared with accelerated dosing of alteplase in the Global Use of Strategies to Open Occluded Coronary Arteries (GUSTO-3).[12]

The RAPID-1 trial demonstrated that reteplase administered as two bolus injections of 10 units each achieved more rapid, complete, and sustained thrombolysis of infarct-related coronary arteries than standard-dose alteplase without an apparent increase in adverse effects.[7] This was an open-label trial enrolling 606 patients from 38 centers in the United States and Europe. Patients with AMI presenting within six hours of symptom onset were randomized to treatment with alteplase 100 mg intravenously over three hours, reteplase as a single 15-unit bolus (10-unit bolus followed by a 5-unit bolus 30 minutes later), or reteplase 10-unit bolus followed by another 10-unit bolus 30 minutes later. Heparin was administered for at least 24 hours with dose adjusted to maintain activated partial thromboplastin time (APTT), and aspirin (200 to 325 mg) was administered prior to the thrombolytic and daily thereafter.

The reteplase group receiving a double bolus of ten units each achieved better 60-minute, 90-minute, and 5- to 14-day complete patency (TIMI [thrombolysis in myocardial infarction] grade 3 flow) than the alteplase group. Patency in the reteplase 10-unit double-bolus group at 60 minutes was equivalent to that of the alteplase group at 90 minutes. Cardiac ejection fraction and regional wall motion in the group receiving a 10-unit double-bolus were superior to the alteplase group at hospital discharge. The other two reteplase regimens produced comparable results. The 30-day mortality was 1.9 percent in the 10-unit double-bolus group and 3.9 percent in the alteplase group. Bleeding risk did not differ between groups.[5,7,13]

Results of studies with accelerated dosing of alteplase prompted an investigation comparing reteplase and front-loaded or accelerated alteplase (the RAPID-2 trial).[7] Patients were recruited from 20 centers in the United States and five in Germany. Patients presenting within 12 hours of ischemic chest pain onset and with electrocardiogram evidence of an AMI were randomized to therapy. The therapy consisted of either two bolus doses of reteplase (ten units administered over two to three minutes) or accelerated alteplase (15 mg bolus, 0.75 mg/kg over 30 minutes with a maximum of 50 mg, then 0.5 mg/kg over 60 minutes with a maximum of 35 mg). A total of 324 patients were enrolled with 165 randomized to reteplase and 159 randomized to alteplase. All patients received intravenous heparin for at least 24 hours with the dose adjusted to APTT and aspirin 160 to 350 mg per day.

Patency was more rapidly and completely achieved in the reteplase group. At 60 minutes, total patency (TIMI grade 2 or 3 flow) was 81.8 percent in the reteplase group compared with 66.1 percent in the alteplase group. Complete patency (TIMI grade 3 flow) was 51.2 percent in the reteplase group compared to 37.4 percent in the alteplase group. Complete reperfusion (TIMI grade 3 flow) at 90 minutes was achieved in 59.9 percent of reteplase-treated patients compared to 45.2 percent of alteplase-treated patients. Total patency (TIMI grade 2 or 3 flow) was higher in the reteplase group; 83.4 percent versus 73.3 percent, respectively.[7] During the first six hours after treatment, fewer patients in the reteplase group (13.6 percent versus 26.5 percent) required additional interventions to restore normal blood flow in the infarct-related coronary artery. Patients in both groups had higher rates of total patency and complete patency when treated within six hours after the onset of symptoms compared to patients treated between six and 12 hours after symptom onset. The investigators also reported that the incidence of reocclusion (9 percent versus 7 percent), the 35-day mortality rates (4.1 percent versus 8.4 percent), the incidence of stroke (1.8 percent versus 2.6 percent), and the rates of hemorrhage did not differ between the groups.[5,14] The reteplase dosing regimen allows for administration of the entire dose within 30 minutes. In contrast, front-loaded alteplase regimens allow only 65 percent of the alteplase dose within 30 minutes. This difference in dosage administration is likely responsible for the more rapid achievement of patency observed with reteplase.

Reteplase was compared to streptokinase in the International Joint Efficacy Comparison of Thrombolytics (INJECT) trial.[9] Patients from 208 centers in nine European countries admitted within 12 hours of AMI onset were randomized to receive either two bolus doses of reteplase (ten units given 30 minutes apart) or streptokinase (1.5 million units given intravenously over 60 minutes). Heparin was administered to 99 percent of patients for at least 24 hours and an initial aspirin dose of 250 to 320 mg was prescribed for 93 percent of patients, followed by 75 to 150 mg daily. A total of 6,010 patients were recruited for the study, with 3,004 randomized to reteplase and 3,006 randomized to streptokinase. By day 35, 9.02 percent of patients in the reteplase group had died compared to 9.53 percent of patients in the streptokinase group. This difference was not significant, but did demonstrate reteplase is equivalent to streptokinase. The odds ratio for reduction in mortality favored reteplase in patients with a history of a previous infarct, and streptokinase in patients with a systolic blood pressure greater than 160 mmHg.

A subgroup analysis of 1,909 patients from Germany enrolled in this study revealed a higher proportion of patients with complete ST segment resolution and a smaller proportion of patients with no ST segment resolution among patients treated with reteplase compared to patients treated with streptokinase.[10] In-hospital strokes occurred in 37 reteplase-treated patients and 30 streptokinase-treated patients. More patients treated with reteplase experienced hemorrhagic strokes. Bleeding events also occurred with a similar frequency in the two groups. The frequency of recurrent myocardial infarction or extension was similar in the two groups, although reductions in atrial fibrillation, asystole, cardiac shock, heart failure, and hypotension were observed in the reteplase group. Statistical analysis revealed that reteplase was equivalent to streptokinase, with a 0.76 probability that reteplase was more effective than streptokinase.[5,9,10,11,15]

Adverse Reactions

Bleeding is the most common adverse effect associated with reteplase. The overall incidence of bleeding in patients treated with reteplase in clinical trials was 21.1 percent. Intracranial hemorrhage occurred in 0.8 percent of patients (23 of 2,965). In comparison, intracranial bleeding was reported in 0.7 percent of patients treated with accelerated dosing of alteplase in clinical trials of alteplase enrolling 10,396 patients, and 1 percent of patients treated with anistreplase in clinical trials of anistreplase enrolling 500 patients.[5,6] Overall, bleeding rates have not differed in clinical trials comparing reteplase with alteplase or streptokinase. It is rare for an allergic or anaphylactoid reaction to occur during reteplase administration. If an anaphylactoid reaction to reteplase occurs, the second bolus should not be administered.[5]

Dosage and Administration

Reteplase is administered as two ten-unit intravenous bolus injections over two minutes. The second bolus is administered 30 minutes after initiation of the first bolus injection. Each injection should be given via an intravenous line in which no other medication is being simultaneously injected or infused.[5] Comparative dosing recommendations with other thrombolytics in the therapy of acute myocardial infarction are summarized in Table 4.2.

No other medication should be added to the injection solution containing reteplase. Heparin and reteplase are incompatible when com-

TABLE 4.2. Comparative FDA-Approved IV Dosages of Thrombolytics Used in AMI Therapy

Thrombolytic	Recommended Dosage
Alteplase	Accelerated regimen
	Patients > 67 kg: 100 mg as a 15 mg bolus, followed by 50 mg infused over the next 30 minutes, and then 35 mg infused over the next 60 minutes
	Patients < 67 kg: 15 mg intravenous bolus, followed by 0.75 mg/kg infused over the next 30 minutes (not to exceed 50 mg), and then 0.5 mg/kg over the next 60 minutes (not to exceed 35 mg)
Reteplase	10 units by intravenous injection over 2 minutes into an intravenous line, followed 30 minutes after the initiation of the first injection by a second 10-unit bolus administered over 2 minutes
Streptokinase	1,500,000 units infused within 60 minutes

Source: Product Information: Alteplase. Genentech, Inc., San Francisco, 1999.

bined in solution and should not be administered simultaneously in the same intravenous line. If reteplase is to be administered through an intravenous line containing heparin, the line should be flushed with normal saline or 5 percent dextrose solution prior to and following reteplase administration.[5]

Reteplase should be reconstituted using the diluent, syringe, needle, and dispensing pin provided. It must be reconstituted with Sterile Water for Injection, USP (without preservatives). Slight foaming upon reconstitution is not unusual, but allowing the vial to stand undisturbed for several minutes will allow dissipation of large bubbles. Reteplase should be used within four hours of reconstitution when stored at 2° to 30°C (36° to 86°F).[5]

LANOTEPLASE

Product Information

Similar to reteplase, lanoteplase is an analog of naturally occurring tissue plasminogen activator (tPA) that rapidly dissolves coronary thrombus. It is currently undergoing clinical trials and has not been approved for treatment.

Pharmacology

Similar to other tPAs, lanoteplase converts plasminogen to the active plasmin, which mediates fibrinolysis. However, unlike other tissue plasminogen activators, lanoteplase can be administered as a single dose.

Clinical Trials

Currently, a large, multinational Phase III trial is being conducted to compare lanoteplase with the current standard, alteplase. In the InTIME II (intravenous nPA for treatment of infarcting myocardium early) trial, 15,078 patients were recruited to compare the 30-day outcomes of MI patients treated with either lanoteplase or alteplase. Patients were randomized to receive either a single IV bolus of lanoteplase 120,000 U/kg or alteplase ≤100 mg as a 90-minute IV infusion. All patients received concomitant antiplatelet treatment of both aspirin and heparin.

Lanoteplase was as effective as alteplase at decreasing 30-day mortality. The 24-hour mortality was slightly better in patients receiving lanoteplase as compared with alteplase. However, patients who received lanoteplase were associated with significantly more intracranial and mild bleeding as compared to alteplase. Intracranial bleeding occurred in 1.13 versus 0.62 percent of lanoteplase and alteplase recipients, respectively (p value ≤ 0.01). Mild bleeding occurred in 19.6 percent versus 14.7 percent of lanoteplase and alteplase recipients, respectively (p value ≤ 0.01). There were no differences between lanoteplase and alteplase in mortality or net clinical outcome at six months (Table 4.3).

TENECTEPLASE

Product Information

Tenecteplase is a genetically engineered variant of alteplase. However, several amino acids were substituted resulting in a modified product with longer half-life and increased fibrin specificity than alteplase. Similar to lanoteplase, tenecteplase is an investigational agent that has not yet been approved for treatment.

Pharmacology

Tenecteplase is a variant of a tPA serine protease that promotes the formation of plasmin. Increased concentrations of plasmin will pro-

TABLE 4.3. Comparison of Lanoteplase and Alteplase

In TIME II Results	Lanoteplase	Alteplase
24-hour mortality (% of patients)	2.39	2.49
30-day mortality (% of patients)	6.77	6.6
Patients with ICH*	0.68	0.4
Patients without ICH	6.11	6.2
% of patients experiencing stroke	1.89	1.52

*Intracranial hemorrhage

mote fibrinolysis, and thus dissolve clots that have formed in coronary arteries.

Clinical Trials

Tenecteplase has been studied in clinical trials involving more than 21,000 patients with acute myocardial infarction. A phase III trial (ASSENT-2) assessed the clinical outcome of tenecteplase.[16] The study recruited and randomized 16,950 patients with acute myocardial infarction who presented within six hours of symptom onset to receive either IV tenecteplase 30-50 mg or IV alteplase as a 90-minute accelerated infusion. The dose of tenecteplase was weight-adjusted; patients received a bolus of 30 to 50 mg depending on body weight.

The 30-day mortality rate was comparable between both tenecteplase (6.15 percent) and alteplase (6.17 percent). However, there was a 2 percent difference in favor of tenecteplase in patients treated within four hours of symptom onset. The rate of total stroke was also similar between the two groups, 1.78 and 1.66 percent with tenecteplase and alteplase, respectively.

Other subgroup analyses found that the incidence of ischemia was lower in women, and in patients younger than 75 years receiving tenecteplase when compared to alteplase. The risks of intracranial hemorrhage were similar among the two treatment groups (0.93 percent versus 0.94 percent of patients, respectively), but the incidence of other bleeding episodes was significantly lower after tenecteplase administration (26 percent versus 28.1 percent, respectively). Transfusion for serious bleeding was significantly less frequent in tenecteplase as compared to alteplase recipients (4.3 percent versus 5.5 percent, respectively). The lower frequency of bleeding may be explained by the increased fibrin specificity of tenecteplase in contrast to alteplase.[16,17]

DORNASE ALFA (Pulmozyme®)

Cystic Fibrosis and Dornase Alfa

Cystic fibrosis (CF) is a lethal disease with a recessive inheritance pattern most common in Caucasians, occurring in approximately one of every 2,500 live white births in the United States.[18] It is characterized by a defect in the chloride transport pump or CF receptor (CTFR). This deficiency in transport of cellular chloride out of epithelial cells is accompanied by a high absorption of intracellular sodium resulting in thick, dehydrated secretions. In the lungs, the net effect is the production of thick, tenacious mucus that impairs pulmonary function and contributes to recurrent or persistent infections. The infected sputum from CF patients contains high levels of DNA liberated from lysed cells.[19]

DNA in sputum binds directly onto protein, thereby preventing leukocyte proteolysis. The viscosity of DNA also reduces the efficacy of various antimicrobials by impeding transport to the affected sites. Aminoglycosides were found to bind onto DNA- and mucin glycopeptide-containing fractions of sputum, thus reducing concentration of the available drug. Dornase alpha reduces viscoelastic properties of CF secretions.[20]

Product Information

Dornase alfa is recombinant human deoxyribonuclease I (rhDNase) that selectively cleaves DNA. The protein is produced by inserting the gene encoding for the native human protein deoxyribonuclease I into CHO, an expression system. rhDNase is purified by tangential flow filtration and column chromatography in which the purified glycoprotein contains 260 amino acids with an approximate molecular weight of 37 kDa.[21] The primary amino acid sequence is identical to that of the native human enzyme. It is approved for use in the adjunctive management of cystic fibrosis to reduce the frequency of respiratory infections requiring antibiotics and to improve pulmonary function.[21]

Each 2.5 mg ampule contains 1.0 mg/mL (2500 U) dornase alfa formulated in 8.77 mg/mL calcium chloride dihydrate, and sterile water for injection. The nominal pH of the solution is 6.3. The formulation contains no preservatives and is stable at room temperature for 24 hours.[21]

Pharmacology

The discovery that deoxyribonuclease I (DNase I) could decrease the viscosity of mucus paved the way for a purified bovine pancreatic

DNase I to be marketed for use in cystic fibrosis patients.[22] Deoxyribonuclease I is naturally found in human serum and in many mammalian and plant tissues. Dornase alfa or recombinant human deoxyribonuclease I (rhDNase I) is an endonuclease that selectively hydrolyzes extracellular DNA into oligonucleotides.[21]

Pharmacokinetics

After 18 CF patients inhaled 2.5 mg dornase alfa, a mean sputum concentration of 3 µg/mL DNase was measured within 15 minutes of administration that declined to 0.6 µg/mL two hours following inhalation. Administered twice a day for six months, no accumulation of dornase alfa was noted.[21]

Clinical Trials

The efficacy of aerosolized dornase alfa has been investigated in a number of trials, involving CF patients with mild to moderate symptoms. Currently, no data are available regarding the efficacy and safety in children younger than five years of age, and limited data are available in patients with severe pulmonary involvement.

Twelve healthy adults and 14 CF patients received aerosolized dornase alfa. Doses ranged from 0.6 mg to 10 mg three times a day, five times a week. In the second week, subjects received a fixed dose of 2 mg, 6 mg, or 10 mg three times daily. Subjects were rechallenged with a single dose 21 days after completion of the initial course. Dornase alfa was well tolerated by both normal subjects and CF patients up to the highest dose. No serious adverse effects were reported for any of the groups. No anaphylactic reactions or anti-DNase antibodies were reported from either group.[23]

Another preliminary study evaluated the effective dose and biochemical efficacy of aerosolized dornase alfa. Sixteen CF patients received either an escalating daily dose (0.1 mg to 20 mg) for seven days or a fixed dosage regimen (20 mg once daily, 10 mg three times a day, or 20 mg twice daily) for six days. No clinically significant adverse effects were reported. An improvement in lung function as measured by increases in FVC (forced vital capacity) and FEV_1 (forced expiratory volume) occurred with all three fixed dosage regimens. The biochemical efficacy was determined by analyzing the DNA chain length in sputum both before and after therapy. Increased amounts of low molecular weight DNA were found after treatment. Following this preliminary study, Hubbard and colleagues evaluated the short-term clinical efficacy of inhaled dornase alfa.[24] Sixteen patients with mild to moderate CF, as defined by a forced vital capacity greater than 40 percent, received 10 mg twice a day for six days. Aerosolized rhDNase significantly improved FEV_1 and FVC (p value < 0.01) relative to baseline levels for days one through six. No changes were noted for other lung measurements such as total lung capacity (TLC), diffusing capacity, and forced expiratory flow during the middle half of FVC (FEF_{50}).[24]

The safety and efficacy of dornase alfa were further evaluated in Phase II trials. Ranasinha and colleagues recruited 71 CF patients with mild to moderate disease to receive either dornase alfa 2.5 mg twice a day or placebo for ten days.[25] The mean percentage change in FEV_1 was 13.3 percent in the dornase alfa group compared to a decline of 0.2 percent in the placebo group (p value < 0.001). The FVC increased 7.2 percent in the treatment group and 2.3 percent in the placebo group. Upon completion of therapy, pulmonary function returned to pretreatment levels.[25]

The efficacy of different doses of dornase alfa was evaluated in another double-blind, placebo-controlled study. One hundred eighty-one outpatients received either 0.6, 2.5, or 10 mg rhDNase twice daily.[26] Baseline characteristics for all treatment groups were similar, except for the 2.5 mg group which reported increased bronchodilator usage during the study (p value = 0.06). By day three, all treatment groups showed significant improvement in FEV_1 relative to baseline (p value < 0.001). However, improvement in FVC was noted only for the 2.5 mg group when compared to placebo (p value < 0.001).[26]

Findings from these clinical trials indicate significant improvement in lung function (~10 to 15 percent above baseline), as measured by FVC, and FEV_1 usually can be seen within the first week of aerosol treatment. Long-term benefit of dornase alfa includes a reduction in the frequency of pulmonary infections requiring intensive antibiotic therapy.[23,24,25,26]

Adverse Reactions

Tolerability data from most studies show dornase alfa to be well tolerated in dosages up to 30 mg per day. There have not been any reports of anaphylaxis or severe allergic responses attributed to dornase alfa. The most commonly associated symptoms associated with dornase alfa have been pharyngitis, voice alteration, and laryngitis.[21]

In a randomized, placebo-controlled clinical trial in patients with FVC 40 percent of predicted, over 600 patients received dornase alfa once or twice daily for six months; most adverse events were not more common with dornase alfa than with placebo and probably reflected the sequelae of the underlying lung disease. In most cases, events that increased were mild, transient in nature, and did not require alterations in dosing. Few patients experienced adverse events resulting in permanent discontinuation from dornase alfa, and the discontinuation rate was similar for placebo (2 percent) and dornase alfa (3 percent).

In a randomized, placebo-controlled trial of patients with advanced disease (FVC < 40 percent of predicted), the safety profile for most adverse events was similar to that reported for the trial in patients with mild to moderate disease.

Dosage and Administration

The recommended dose of dornase alfa for most cystic fibrosis patients (older than five years of age) is 2.5 mg inhaled once daily using a recommended nebulizer. Some patients may benefit from twice-daily administration.[21] Recommended nebulizers include disposable jet nebulizer Hudson T Up-Draft II; disposable jet nebulizer Marquest Acorn II in conjunction with a Pulmo-Aide compressor; and reusable PARI LC Jet nebulizer in conjunction with the PARI PRONEB compressor. The safety and efficacy of dornase alfa use in children younger than five years old has not been established.

NOTES

1. Product Information: Alteplase. San Francisco: Genentech, Inc, 1999.
2. Clinical Pharmacology, Product Information: Alteplase. San Francisco: Genentech, Inc., 1999.
3. The National Institute of Neurological Disorders and Stroke, rt-PA Stroke Study Group. Tissue plasminogen activator for acute ischemic stroke. *N Engl J Med* 1995;333:1581-1587.
4. Anonymous. Six-month survival in 20,891 patients with acute myocardial infarction randomized between alteplase and streptokinase with or without heparin.

GISSI-2 and International Study Group. Gruppo Italiano per lo Studio della Sopravvivenza nell 'Infarto. *European Heart Journal* 1992;13:1692-1697.

5. Boehringer Mannheim. Package literature for *Retavase*. Malvern, PA: Centocor, Inc.

6. Denniston PL. *Physician's GenRx 1997.* Riverside, CT: Denniston Publishing, Inc., 1996.

7. Weaver WD. Results of the RAPID 1 and RAPID 2 thrombolytic trials in acute myocardial infarction. *Eur Heart J* 1996;17:14-20.

8. Stringer KA. Biochemical and pharmacologic comparison of thrombolytic agents. *Pharmacotherapy* 1996;16(5, Pt 2):119S-126S.

9. Hampton JR. Mega-trials and equivalence trials: Experience from the INJECT study. *Eur Heart J* 1996;17:28-34.

10. International Joint Efficacy Comparison of Thrombolytics. Randomized, double-blind comparison of reteplase double-bolus administration with streptokinase in acute myocardial infarction (INJECT): Trial to investigate equivalence. *Lancet* 1995; 346:329-336.

11. Armstrong PW. Perspectives gained from large-scale thrombolytic comparative trials. *Eur Heart J* 1996;17:9-13.

12. Amsterdam EA. Controlled trials comparing reteplase with alteplase and streptokinase in patients with acute myocardial infarction. *Pharmacotherapy* 1996;16(5, Pt 2):137S-140S.

13. Smalling RW, Bode C, Kalbfleisch J, Limbourg P, Forycki F, Habib G, Feldman R, Hohnloser S, Seals A. More rapid, complete, and stable coronary thrombolysis with bolus administration of reteplase compared with alteplase infusion in acute myocardial infarction. *Circulation* 1995;91:2725-2732.

14. Bode C, Smalling RW, Berg G, Burnett C, Lorch G, Kalfleisch JM, Cheroff R, Christie LG, Feldman RL, Seals A. Randomized comparison of coronary thrombolysis achieved with double-bolus reteplase (recombinant plasminogen activator) and front-loaded, accelerated alteplase (recombinant tissue plasminogen activator) in patients with acute myocardial infarction. *Circulation* 1996;94:891-898.

15. Schroder R, Wegscheider K, Schroder K, Dissmann R, Meyer-Sabellek W. Extent of early ST segment elevation resolution: A strong predictor of outcome in patients with acute myocardial infarction and a sensitive measure to compare thrombolytic regimens. A substudy of the International Joint Efficacy Comparison of Thrombolytics (INJECT) Trial. *J Am Coll Cardiol* 1995;26:1657-1664.

16. Van de Werf F, Barron HV, Armstrong PW, Granger CB, Berioli S, Barbash G, Pehrsson K, Verheugt FW, Meyer J, Betriu A. Incidence and predictors of bleeding events after fibrinolytic therapy with fibrin-specific agents: A comparison of TNK-tPA and rt-PA. *European Heart Journal* 2001;72(24):2221-2223.

17. Neuhaus K-L. A phase three trial of novel bolus thrombolytic lanoteplase (nPA): Intravenous or PA for treatment of infarcting myocardium early (In Time-II). *J Am Coll Cardiol* 1999;33(February).

18. Knowles MR. New therapies for cystic fibrosis: Introduction. *Chest* 1995; 107:59S-60S.

19. Raskin P. Bronchospasm after inhalation of pancreatic dornase. *Am Rev Respir Dis* 1968;98:697-698.

20. Spier R, Witebsky E, Paine J. Aerosolized pancreatic dornase and antibiotics in pulmonary infections. *JAMA* 1961;178:878-886.

21. Package insert: Pulmozyme (Dornase alfa recombinant inhalation solution). Genentech, San Francisco, CA, 1994.

22. Shak S, Capon DJ, Hellmiss R, Warsters SA, Baker CL. Recombinant human DNase I reduces the viscosity of cystic fibrosis sputum. *Proc Natl Acad Sci USA* 1990;87:9188-9192.

23. Aitken ML, Burke W, McDonald G, Shak S, Montgomery AB, Smith A. Effect of inhaled recombinant DNase on pulmonary function in normal and cystic fibrosis patients: Phase I study. *JAMA* 1992;267:1947-1951.

24. Hubbard RC, McElvaney NG, Birrer P, Shak S, Robinson WW, Jolley C, Wu M, Chernick MS, Crystal RG. A preliminary study of aerosolized recombinant human deoxyribonuclease I in the treatment of cystic fibrosis. *N Engl J Med* 1992; 326:812-815.

25. Ranasinha C, Assoufi B, Shak S, Christiansen D, Fuchs H, Empey D, Geddes D, Hodson M. Efficacy and safety of short-term administration of aerosolized recombinant human DNase I in adults with stable stage cystic fibrosis. *Lancet* 1993;342:199-202.

26. Ramsey BW, Astley SJ, Aitken ML, Burke W, Colin AA, Dorkin HL, Eisenberg JD, Gibson RL, Harwood IR, Schidlow DV. Efficacy and safety of short-term administration of aerosolized recombinant human deoxyribonuclease in patients with cystic fibrosis. *Am Rev Respir Dis* 1993;148:145-151.

Chapter 5

Cytokines

Stan G. Louie
Parul Patel

INTRODUCTION

Cytokines are defined as cellular hormones that require receptor binding onto specific receptors to elicit cellular responses. Although the majority of these responses are stimulatory in nature, cytokines can also induce inhibitory responses. This chapter focuses on the various hematopoietic growth factors that influence the maturation and activation of circulating cells which are found in the blood (Figure 5.1). These factors are segmented into either lymphoid or myeloid factors. Lymphoid factors include interleukin and the interferon family of factors. In contrast, the myeloid factors include colony-stimulating factors.[1]

After the discovery and characterization of these cytokines, a number of them were cloned and expressed using recombinant technology. The ability to produce large quantities of these factors allowed for the creation of immunotherapy, in which cytokines are given to enhance the immune response to various conditions.

INTERLEUKIN-2

Interleukin-2 (IL-2) is a T-lymphocyte cytokine that enhances cellular immunity, particularly cytotoxic T-lymphocyte (CTLs) and natural killer cell (NK) activities. IL-2 can also stimulate B-lymphocytes and increase the expression of various cytokines such as tumor necrosis factor (TNF), interleukin-1 (IL-1), interferon-γ (IFN-γ), and granulocyte macrophage colony-stimulating factor (GM-CSF).[1] In its

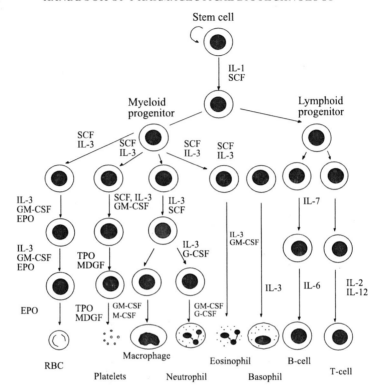

FIGURE 5.1. Hematopoietic paradigm

natural form, IL-2 is a 133 amino acid glycoprotein with varying degrees of glycosylation. It is the natural ligand of IL-2 receptor (IL-2R), which is present on both T-lymphocytes and natural killer cells.

Aldesleukin (Proleukin®)

Product Information

Aldesleukin is indicated for use in patients with metastatic renal cell carcinoma and metastatic melanoma. Also known as recombinant human IL-2 (rhIL-2), aldesleukin is produced by insertion of plasmid containing recombinant IL-2 gene into an *E. coli* expression system.[2] The IL-2 gene has been modified, so that the recombinant protein product is identical to natural IL-2 with the exception of a serine residue substitution for cysteine on position 125. In addition, the recombinant product lacks an alanine residue on the N-terminus. The molecular weight for this unglycosylated rhIL-2 is 15.3 kDa, and has the same binding affinity as natural IL-2.[2]

Pharmacokinetics

As is any biological agent, rhIL-2 is rapidly distributed and eliminated (Table 5.1). The distribution half-life ($t_{1/2\alpha}$) was found to be 13.4 minutes, while the elimination half-life ($t_{1/2\beta}$) was 85 minutes.[3] Five minutes after an intravenous injection of rhIL-2, only 30 percent of the injected dose remained in the plasma compartment, suggesting that rhIL-2 rapidly distributes into visceral organs such as the liver, kidney, and lungs. However, the volume of distribution is reported to be 4.3 L, whereas the area under the curve is 14,500 units/mL per minute per dose. In addition, rhIL-2 is reported to have a rapid clearance of 117 mL/min.[3]

Clinical Uses

Renal cell carcinoma. The primary clinical use of aldesleukin or rhIL-2 is to stimulate T-lymphocytes to attack any neoplastic growth. When rhIL-2 is administered as a continuous infusion, a dramatic reduction in tumor burden is noted. The mechanism of antitumor effect has been attributed to expansion and activation of cytotoxic T-lymphocytes (CTLs) and natural killer cells (NK).

Stimulated CTLs and NK cells can also be expanded and maintained in culture in the presence of rhIL-2. In initial clinical trials, lymphocytes were harvested from the patients' blood and expanded

TABLE 5.1. Pharmacokinetic Parameters of rhIL-2

Pharmacokinetic Parameter	Values
$t_{1/2\alpha}$	13.4 min
$t_{1/2\beta}$	85 min
AUC	14,500 units/mL per min per dose
Vd	4.3 L

in culture or ex vivo. The expanded lymphocytes were reinfused back into the patient along with high doses of rhIL-2 (>100,000 units/kg every 8 h). This treatment was able to produce a 90 percent response among patients with disseminated renal cell carcinoma.[4] These responses rates were amazing because these patients had already failed other conventional and salvage therapies. However, the response rates against other tumor types were less dramatic; clinical responses were only 50 percent in patients with metastatic melanoma, and 30 percent in patients with metastatic colon cancer.[4]

Due to the high cost of maintaining and expanding lymphocytes in culture, the efficacy of activated lymphocytes in combination with high doses of rhIL-2 was compared to high dose rhIL-2 alone. Initially, patients receiving both rhIL-2 stimulated lymphocytes with high dose rhIL-2 had better survival rates than those receiving rhIL-2 alone.[5] However, long-term survival was not significantly different when rhIL-2 with activated lymphocytes was compared to rhIL-2 alone. Thus, high dose IL-2 was shown to be equivalent to stimulated lymphocytes combined with high dose rhIL-2 with no difference in clinical outcome.[5]

Human immunodeficiency virus. IL-2 is a T-cell growth factor that has been described to have antiviral activity against Epstein-Barr virus (EBV), cytomegalovirus (CMV), and human immunodeficiency virus (HIV). T-cells isolated from HIV-infected patients were found to have lowered levels of IL-2 expression when compared to non-infected individuals. The reduction in IL-2 expression may lower the capacity to expand T-cells, thus accounting for reduced antigenic stimulation response. Furthermore, prolonged IL-2 deficiency may explain why T-cells from HIV patients have increased levels of cellular suicide or apoptotic activity.

rhIL-2 was first employed in HIV-infected patients in an effort to boost the declining immune system. However, despite over ten years of experience, there is still no conclusive evidence regarding its benefit in HIV-infected patients. Another controversy concerns IL-2's ability to stimulate HIV proliferation. When rhIL-2 is administered without antiretroviral agents, there is an increased level of HIV proliferation. This is attributed to rhIL-2's ability to stimulate activity of the HIV transactivatory *(tat)* gene. Conversely, rhIL-2 is also able to expand CD4 cells, which can increase the number of potential reservoirs available for HIV infections. In addition, IL-2 can induce expression of other inflammatory factors, such as interleukin-1 (IL-1) and tumor necrosis factor (TNF), which can in turn activate *tat* expression.

The potential of rhIL-2 to stimulate HIV proliferation suggests that any trial involving IL-2 in HIV must also include antiretroviral agents. Despite the addition of zidovudine (AZT), the combination of IL-2 and AZT did not demonstrate significant clinical improvements. This may be due to the short duration of AZT therapy.

When high doses of rhIL-2 were given as an intermittent continuous infusion in HIV patients with antiretroviral agents, an increased expression of interleukin-2 receptor (IL-2R) was noted. One clinical effect was the acceleration of CD4 cell recovery, in which 6 out of 10 patients had increased CD4 levels that were 50 percent above their baseline levels. These clinical benefits were seen in patients with an intact immune system, with baseline CD4 levels above 200 cells/mm^3. However, only 2 out of 10 patients responded to rhIL-2 therapy when baseline CD4 counts were below 200 cells/mm^3. In contrast, no clinical improvement was seen in patients with baseline CD4 counts below 100 cells/mm^3.

Smaller doses of rhIL-2 were employed in combination with zidovudine due to concerns that high levels of rhIL-2 may be more effective in stimulating HIV proliferation. Furthermore, lower levels of rhIL-2 are required to increase NK cell expression of IL-2R. Smaller doses of rhIL-2 were also associated with reduction in the severity and incidence of adverse effects.

Adverse Reactions

Tolerance of IL-2 therapy is proportional to dose. High-dose therapy is characterized as doses greater than 100,000 units/kg every eight hours and is associated with significant adverse effects. These side effects are related to rhIL-2-induced leaky capillary syndrome, in which the activated lymphocytes break through the vasculature to gain access to the tumor. Vascular breakdown permits intravascular contents to leak out into the extracellular space.

Intravascular fluid loss manifests clinically as hypotension, peripheral edema, renal failure, and pleural effusion. Patients receiving 600,000 units/kg of rhIL-2 every eight hours may require treatment with β-adrenergic agonists, such as dopamine, dobutamine, or epinephrine, to maintain blood pressure. At times, it may also be necessary to add vasoconstricting α-adrenergic agonist agents, such as phenylephrine along with β-agonists to maintain blood pressure.[4]

When lymphocytes extravasate into kidneys, renal insufficiency may develop resulting in an increased blood urea nitrogen (BUN) and serum creatinine. In contrast, lymphocyte extravasation in the liver may result in liver damage, manifesting in elevations of liver enzymes such as transaminase and alkaline phosphatase.

Fluid accumulation in other areas may manifest as peripheral edema, and pleural and pericardial effusion. When left untreated, these adverse effects may lead to pulmonary congestion and even congestive heart failure. Progressive intravascular fluid loss requires cardiac compensation, which may lead to ventricular tachycardia. If ventricular tachycardia continues, reduced myocardial perfusion can lead to cellular necrosis, causing ischemia and ultimately resulting in congestive heart failure.

rhIL-2 is also associated with the development of flulike syndromes. This adverse effect may be caused by the production of other inflammatory mediators such as IL-1, TNF, IL-6, and IFN-γ via rhIL-2 stimulation. Patients receiving low-dose rhIL-2 therapy exhibit this flulike syndrome and complain of arthralgias, myalgias, chills, and fever.[2]

A number of dose-related toxicities are associated with IL-2 infusion (Table 5.2). These include vital signs (blood pressure, temperature, respiratory rate, and pulse), laboratory values measuring serum creatinine, BUN, and liver enzymes (i.e., alkaline phosphatase, alanine transferase, asparate transferase, bilirubin, and lactate dehydrogenase).[2] Blood oxygenation should also be closely monitored because an increase in pulmonary fluids can reduce oxygenation capabilities. The amount of fluids that the patient receives and eliminates and a measure of weight gain are good indicators of fluid retention. When IL-2 is stopped, all of the aforementioned adverse effects will ameliorate with time.[2]

INTERLEUKIN-11

The wide use of cytotoxic chemotherapy agents has led to a dramatic rise in hematological toxicities in cancer patients. Among

TABLE 5.2. Toxicities of IL-2

Dosage	Effect
High dose of IL-2	Hypotension
	Renal dysfunction
	Peripheral edema
	Epidermis exfoliation
	Retina detachment
	Pulmonary and pericardial effusion
Low dose of IL-2	Chills
	Fever
	Malaise
	Myalgias
	Arthralgias

them, thrombocytopenia has become an increasingly common dose-related side effect.[6,7] In 1992, 8.3 million units of platelets were transfused in the United States, nearly three times the volume in 1980.[8] Until now, only labor-intensive, donated platelets have been used to treat chemotherapy-induced thrombocytopenia. This treatment modality is extremely expensive, time-consuming, and associated with an increased risk of infectious agent transmission.[7]

Interleukin-11 (IL-11) is a cytokine and a member of growth factors including interleukin-3 (IL-3) and granulocyte macrophage colony-stimulating factor (GM-CSF), which plays a role in thrombocytopoiesis.[9] IL-11 was first isolated from the stromal cells found in the bone marrow of primates.[10] In vitro, IL-11 increases the number and maturation of megakaryocytes that will form platelets.[10,11,12] IL-11 also augments the effects of IL-3 and GM-CSF to promote the proliferation of a number of hematopoietic cells.[13]

In addition to its thrombopoietic properties, IL-11 exhibits potent anti-inflammatory activity by down-regulating the expression of pro-inflammatory cytokines such as tumor necrosis factor, IL-1, and IL-12.[14] Due to an ability to stimulate platelet production, a recombinant form of IL-11 has been developed to treat thrombocytopenia on a much larger scale.

Oprelvekin (Neumega®)

Product Information

Oprelvekin or rhIL-11 is indicated for the prevention of severe thrombocytopenia and reduction of platelet transfusions in patients with nonmyeloid malignancies who are treated with cytotoxic chemotherapy. Oprelvekin is produced by inserting the cDNA encoding for IL-11 into *E. coli*. Since the inserted gene lacks the code for an N-terminal proline, the purified protein consists of 177 amino acids. The recombinant is missing a proline residue; however, it has the identical biological activity as native IL-11.[9]

Pharmacokinetics

After an oprelvekin dose of 50 μg/kg, the Cmax was determined to occur three hours after infusion, with a level of 19 ng/ml. The bioavailability of oprelvekin is 80 percent, and the half-life was demonstrated to be seven hours. [6,15] Oprelvekin is thought to be metabolized primarily in the liver. The mean clearance of rhIL-11 was found to be 40 percent lower in patients with severe renal impairment; however, the terminal half-life was found to be similar to those with normal renal function.[9] The clearance of oprelvekin was found to be 1.2 to 1.8 times higher in children when compared to adults.[9] The onset of biological response was five to nine days after the first injection, with increasing effect for up to seven days after the last injection. However, platelets returned to near baseline values after discontinuation of therapy.[6]

Clinical Trials

In an open-label, nonrandomized phase I trial, 16 female patients with breast cancer were randomized to receive four different dosage levels of recombinant IL-11 before and after the first round of chemotherapy.[6] The cohorts, consisting of three to five women each, were assigned to receive either 10, 25, 50, or 75 μg/kg per day of rhIL-11 subcutaneously for 14 days, followed by a 14-day washout period. After this initial 28-day cycle, patients received up to four monthly treatments of chemotherapy consisting of doxorubicin and cyclophosphamide. The patients then received their assigned dose of rhIL-

11 for 12 days following the chemotherapy. Platelet increases of 76, 93, 108, and 185 percent were seen with the 10, 25, 50, and 75 μg/kg dose levels, respectively, during the first prechemotherapy phase of treatment. During this phase, a 20 percent decrease in hematocrit was seen in all dosage arms, suggesting that rhIL-11 had no effect on chemotherapy-induced anemia. During the second postchemotherapy phase of the trial, the median platelet counts for patients receiving doses > 25 μg/kg per day were significantly higher than patients receiving only 10 μg/kg per day.[6] Overall, the study suggests that doses of > 25 μg/kg per day will significantly reduce the impact of chemotherapy-induced thrombocytopenia in these patients.

A randomized, placebo-controlled, double-blinded study compared two doses of oprelvekin to placebo in 93 patients receiving one cycle of chemotherapy who had already been transfused with platelets during their previous chemotherapy cycle.[7] Oprelvekin or placebo were given as daily subcutaneous injections starting the day following the completion of chemotherapy. The regimen was continued for 14 to 21 days or until platelet counts increased above 100,000 cells. Patients were assigned to receive either 25 μg/kg or 50 μg/kg of rhIL-11 or placebo. In the group that received rhIL-11 at 50 μg/kg, eight (30 percent) did not require additional platelet transfusions in comparison to one (4 percent) with placebo. For those receiving 25 μg/kg of oprelvekin, 5 out of 28 (18 percent) avoided transfusions.[7] The study demonstrates that oprelvekin at doses of 50 μg/kg per day significantly reduced the need for further platelet transfusions in patients receiving dose-intensive chemotherapy.

Adverse Reactions

The most commonly reported adverse reaction in patients receiving oprelvekin is a generalized edema ranging from 40 to 60 percent depending on the study. This reaction is believed to be a result of sodium retention associated with the use of this drug.[7,9] The increase in plasma volume also leads to a dilutional decrease in hemoglobin and hematocrit concentrations. Other adverse reactions include arthralgias, myalgias, headache, tachycardia, and palpitation.[6,7] Less common reactions include papilledema, dyspnea, and pleural effusions. Rare reports of fatal hypokalemia in two patients receiving 50 μg/kg per day, and a 1 percent incidence of the development of rhIL-11 antibodies were documented.[9]

Dosage and Administration

A baseline complete blood count should be performed prior to chemotherapy and start of oprelvekin therapy. From there, platelet counts should be assessed until adequate recovery has occurred (i.e., > 50,000/mm^3).[9] The recommended dose of oprelvekin for adults is 50 µg/kg given daily as subcutaneous injections for 10 to 21 days or until platelets rise above 50,000/mm^3 postnadir. For children, the recommended dose is 75 to 100 µg/kg.[9] The treatment should be started six to 24 hours after the last dose of chemotherapy, and discontinued at least two days prior to the next chemotherapy session. Oprelvekin can be administered subcutaneously in either the abdomen, thigh, hip, or upper arm.[9]

Each vial must be reconstituted with 1 mL of the supplied sterile water for injection. The solution should be reconstituted carefully, avoiding any rigorous shaking or agitation. The resultant solution contains 5 mg/mL of rhIL-11. The appropriate amount of drug should be withdrawn from the vial and injected immediately. Any unused portion should be discarded.[9] The final solution should be used within three hours of reconstitution. The solution should not be frozen or shaken rigorously. The lyophilized powder and sterile water for injection should be stored at 2° to 8°C (36° to 46°F).[9]

INTERFERONS

Interferons (IFNs) are a family of naturally occurring glycoproteins that are secreted by the body in response to antigenic intrusion, especially viral infections. IFNs exert their biological activities by inducing the expression of antiviral proteins (Figure 5.2). The transcription of antiviral proteins begins with IFN binding onto a membrane receptor, which activates a series of intracellular signals and ultimately leads to enhanced expression of interferon-induced genes. These genes encode for proteins that include 2'-5'-oligoadenylate synthetase and protein kinases, which have antiviral activity.[16]

IFNs are classified into three major categories depending on the molecule's cellular origin of the molecules. Interferon-α (IFN-α) is

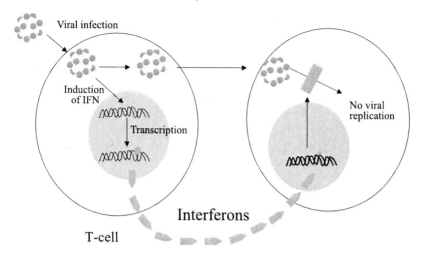

FIGURE 5.2. Mechanism of action of IFN

in a family of IFNs that is derived from leukocytes. In contrast, interferon-β (IFN-β) and interferon-γ (IFN-γ) are produced by fibroblasts and lymphocytes, respectively. IFNs have also been classified in terms of their receptor binding and are classified as either type I or II. Both IFN-α and IFN-β bind onto type I receptors, and are referred to as type I IFNs. Since IFN-α and -β bind onto the same receptor, both seem to exert similar biological activity. IFN-γ is the only IFN that binds onto type II receptors, and thus is classified as a type II IFN.[16]

Physiologically, IFNs are produced in response to foreign intrusion, such as in the case of a viral infection. When blood levels of IFNs are sufficiently elevated, lymphocyte expansion and activation of cellular immunity is observed. Although IFNs can activate and stimulate myriad cells, its most prominent biological activity is activation of CTLs. Another biological activity associated with IFN activation includes the induction of target cell expression of major histocompatibility complex (MHC) class I antigen, enabling immune cells to more easily recognize them as foreign cells. IFNs have also been shown to increase (1) expansion of NK cells, (2) cytotoxic activity of CTLs, (3) phagocytic activity of macrophages, and (4) antibody-dependent cell-mediated cytotoxicity (ADCC).[16]

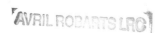

Interferon-α

There are at least 25 different naturally occurring species of interferon-α (IFN-α), all of which generally have either 165 or 166 amino acid residues in its polypeptide backbone.[17] The family of IFN-α is highly conserved and is relatively species specific. Currently, there are four commercially available IFN-α products in Europe; only three compounds are available in the United States (Table 5.3). The approved indications of IFN-α vary with the product. The range of indications includes the treatment of hairy cell leukemia, multiple myeloma, malignant melanoma, chronic myelogenous leukemia (CML), condylomata acuminata, AIDS-related Kaposi's sarcoma (AIDS-KS), and chronic hepatitis (B and C) infections (Box 5.1).

Many of these conditions have been associated with viral infections (Table 5.4). Hairy cell leukemia is associated with infection by human T-lymphotropic virus-II (HTLV-II). Condylomata acuminata or venereal wart has been linked to infection with human papilloma virus (HPV). AIDS-related Kaposi's sarcoma and multiple myeloma have been associated with the same virus family—herpes virus-VIII (HSV-8).[16]

These viruses are thought to be oncogenic or capable of transforming infected cells into malignant cells. The mechanism by which

TABLE 5.3. Commercially Available Interferon-α

Biological Designation	Trade Name	Indications
Interferon-α 2a*	Roferon	Hairy cell leukemia, hepatitis C virus, chronic myelogous leukemia, multiple myeloma, melanoma
Interferon-α 2b*	Intron A	Hairy cell leukemia, hepatitis B and C viruses, AIDS-related Kaposi's sarcoma, chronic myelogous leukemia (CML), condylomata acuminata (venereal warts), multiple myeloma, melanoma
Interferon-α N1	Alferon-N1	
Interferon-α consensus*	Imfergen	Hepatitis C virus

*Available in the United States

BOX 5.1. Clinical Uses for Interferon-α

Chronic myelogous leukemia
Human papilloma virus
Acute T-cell leukemia and lymphoma
Multiple myeloma
Nasopharyngeal carcinoma
AIDS-related Kaposi's sarcoma
Malignant melanoma
Renal cell carcinoma

TABLE 5.4. Virally Linked Tumors

Disorders	Associated Virus
Hairy cell leukemia	Human T-lymphotropic virus-II (HTLV-II)
Multiple myeloma	Human herpesvirus-VIII (HSV-VIII) or Kaposi's sarcoma associated herpesvirus (KSHV)
AIDS-related Kaposi's sarcoma	Human herpesvirus-VIII (HSV-VIII) or Kaposi's sarcoma associated herpesvirus (KSHV)
Condylomata acuminata	Human papilloma virus (HPV)
Hepatocellular carcinoma	Hepatitis B (HBV) and C viruses (HCV)

IFN-α exerts its biological activity is related in its ability to inhibit virus proliferation.[17] The inhibition of viral proliferation will ultimately block cellular transformation and/or expression of growth factors that may promote tumor development. Other antitumor properties ascribed to IFN-α include inhibition of new capillary formation or angiogenesis.[18] Proliferating tissues require nutrients to sustain growth, which is attained through neovascularization. IFN-α's ability to inhibit angiogenesis has been one reason it is capable of inhibiting Kaposi's sarcoma proliferation. Furthermore, IFN-α has been shown to inhibit virally induced expression of cytokines, such as interleukin-6 (IL-6) and oncostatin-M, which are mitogens of various malignancies such as AIDS-KS and multiple myeloma.[16]

Interferon-α 2a, Recombinant (Roferon®)

Product information. Interferon-α 2a (IFN-α 2a or Roferon) is approved for the treatment of chronic hepatitis C, hairy cell leukemia, and AIDS-related Kaposi's sarcoma. Using recombinant technology, the natural IFN-α gene derived from leukocytes was altered and recombined into a plasmid. The recombinant plasmids were then incorporated into *E. coli* expression systems.[19] The protein by-product is a 19 kDa nonglycosylated protein with an amino acid sequence identical to the naturally occurring IFN-α, with the exception of a lysine substitution on the twenty-third position.

Interferon-α 2b, Recombinant (Intron A®)

Product information. Interferon-α 2b (IFN-α 2b or Intron A) is indicated for use in conjunction with chemotherapy in patients with follicular lymphoma. This product is similar to IFN-α 2a since they are both produced through recombinant technology.[20] A comparison between the two products is outlined in Table 5.5. Both molecules have 165 amino acids in their protein backbones with a deletion of an amino acid on the forty-fourth position. The major difference between the two is that IFN-α 2a has lysine on the twenty-third position, whereas IFN-α 2b has an arginine residue at that position. This accounts for the difference in molecular weights between the two recombinant products.

Similar to IFN-α 2a, IFN-α 2b is produced by the insertion of a recombinant plasmid containing the modified IFN-α gene. Since the expression system used is *E. coli*, the final recombinant product is unglycosylated.

Comparison of Interferon-α 2a with Interferon-α 2b

Controversy surrounds both of these products. This controversy revolves around the effect of one amino acid difference on the twenty-third position. Some have argued that the difference between IFN-α 2a and IFN-α 2b is in antigenicity. The formation of anti-IFN-α antibodies has been associated with lowered biological potency. However, evidence indicates that a change in amino acid on the

TABLE 5.5. A Comparison of Interferon-α 2a and Interferon-α 2b

Category	Roferon	Intron A
Indications	Chronic hepatitis C, hairy cell leukemia, AIDS-KS, CML	Chronic hepatitis C and B, hairy cell leukemia, AIDS-KS, malignant melanoma, and condylomata acuminata.
Expression system	*E. coli*	*E. coli*
Specific activity	2 × 108 IU/mg protein	2 × 108 IU/mg protein
Molecular weight	19,000 daltons	19,271 daltons
Amino acid substitution on 23rd residue	Lysine	Arginine
Purification procedure	Affinity column	Physicochemical separation
Formulation	Solution containing: NaCl, polysorbate 80, benzyl alcohol, and ammonium acetate	Solution containing: NaCl, NaH_2PO4, Na_2HPO4, EDTA, polysorbate 80, and *m*-cresol

twenty-third position is neither involved in receptor binding nor antigenicity.[17]

Both IFN-α 2a and IFN-α 2b have identical specific biological activities, suggesting that any modification at the twenty-third position has no effect on receptor binding or the ability to activate signal transduction.[19,20] It remains undetermined whether clinically important differences in therapeutic and/or toxicological profiles may exist between these two products.

Interferon-α Consensus

Interferon-α con-1 (IFN-α con-1) is the newest entry into the marketplace.[21] This product is unlike the other two recombinant products in two significant ways. First, the polypeptide backbone consists of 166 amino acids. Second, and more important, IFN-α con-1 is not the result of a single amino acid modification from a naturally occurring IFN gene. Rather, IFN-α con-1 is an amalgamation of sequences from IFN-α subtypes. This recombinant product differs from other

IFN-α in 20 of 166 amino acids, retaining 80 percent homology. IFN-α con-1 is a synthetically constructed sequence that was expressed in an *E. coli* system, which yields a product weighing 19 kDa.[21]

Pharmacokinetics

The pharmacokinetic parameters of the IFN-α commercial products are similar and are summarized in Table 5.6. There is little difference whether the product is a mixture or pure recombinant product.

After an intramuscular or subcutaneous injection of IFN-α 2a, the fraction of drug absorbed exceeds 80 percent. The peak concentrations achieved after a dose of 36 million units (MU), either through an intravenous (IV), intramuscular (IM), or subcutaneous (SC) route, are 2320, 340, and 290 units/mL, respectively. The time to peak concentration was 15 to 60 minutes when IFN-α was administered as an IV bolus. When the dose was given as an IM or SC injection, the time to peak was significantly slower, where maximum concentration was reached one to eight hours after the administration of the dose.[16,20]

The total body clearance was 0.6 to 1.4 mL/min per kg. However, half-life differed between healthy individuals and those with disseminated malignancies. Healthy individuals had an average half-life of

TABLE 5.6. Pharmacokinetics of Interferon-α

Pharmacokinetic Parameter	Values
Fraction absorbed	80% (SC or IM)
	100% (IV)
Peak concentration (Dose of 36 MU)	2,320 units/mL (IV)
	340 units/mL (IM)
	290 units/mL (SC)
Time to peak	15-60 min (IV)
	1-8 h (IM)
	6-8 h (SC)
Half-life ($t_{1/2}$)	5.1 h (healthy volunteers)
	0.75-2 h (disseminated cancer patients)
Total body clearance	0.6-1.4 mL/min per kg

5.1 hours, whereas patients with disseminated cancers had a shorter half-life (0.75 to 2 hours).

Clinical Uses

Chronic hepatitis B. Hepatitis B virus (HBV) is a hepadnavirus that is primarily transmitted through infected blood supply, intimate contact with infected individuals, and maternal transfer to fetus. HBV has an incubation period that ranges from two to three months. Following viral entry into the body, the incubation period can range from two to four months. Acute infection can lead to liver failure; approximately 1 percent of infected patients develop hepatic cirrhosis. Fortunately, the majority of these patients are asymptomatic and do not have signs of disease. However, asymptomatic patients can develop chronic infections capable of viral transmission and are frequently referred to as carriers. Chronic HBV infections affect approximately 2 percent of infected patients and have been associated with an increased risk of developing primary hepatocellular carcinoma.

IFN-α 2b is the only IFN that is approved for the treatment of adults with chronic active HBV infection. Patients who are undergoing IFN therapy should show evidence of chronic infection with HBV by the presence of the hepatitis B surface antigen (HBsAg), circulating hepatitis B "e" (HBeAg) antigen, and polymerase chain reactions (PCR) positive for the HBV DNA. Other important laboratory tests should include serum aminotransferase activity such as alanine transferase (ALT) and aspartate transferase (AST). Despite these tests, it is necessary to confirm HBV infection by ascertaining a liver biopsy.

Patients who do not qualify for IFN therapy include those with severe, decompensated liver disease (e.g., encephalopathy, ascites, high bilirubin, prolonged prothrombin time) and those with acute active HBV infections. The recommended dosage of rhIFN-α 2b for the treatment of chronic HBV is 5,000,000 units (5 MU) daily, which is administered as either an SC or IM injection. Although lower doses of IFN-α 2b can be used, it was found that response is dose dependent. The recommended duration of therapy is a minimum of 16 weeks with evidence suggesting that prolonged therapy (one year or longer) may decrease the incidence of HBV relapse.[20]

A meta-analysis of various trials showed that 45 percent of patients with chronic hepatitis B treated with IFN-α 2b were able to decrease the level of viral replication and reduce serum HBeAg. One year after treatment, 8 percent of the patients were found to have no evidence of HBsAg, which is drastically better than the case in untreated patients (1 percent free of HBsAg).[20]

Chronic hepatitis C. Hepatitis C, or non-A, non-B hepatitis, virus (HCV) is an RNA virus with a lipid envelope that can cause liver cirrhosis, hepatic failure, and hepatocellular carcinoma. Its mode of transmission is similar to HBV and HIV, namely through infected blood products, intimate contact with infected individuals, and maternal transfer to the uninfected fetus. This flavidiviridae virus does not have a DNA intermediate, thus is unable to integrate into the host genome. However, despite this feature, HCV has a chronic phase that is difficult to eliminate.

Following initial infection, the incubation period of HCV has a range of 45 to 55 days. Unlike other hepatitis infections, the acute phase of HCV is generally mild and manifests as generalized malaise and the development of flulike symptoms without the evidence of jaundice or other hepatic injury. Although rare, fulminant HCV can occur and is associated with a high mortality.

If left untreated, approximately 90 percent of the patients with HCV will develop persistent infection. Forty percent of these patients will develop no symptoms, and approximately 60 percent will develop chronic hepatitis 10 to 20 years after the initial infection. This long duration to cellular injury allows the infection to progress unchecked without treatment.

The most frequently encountered clinical complication associated with chronic HCV infection is hepatic cirrhosis, which occurs in 20 to 50 percent of patients. Other complications include increased risk of developing hepatocellular carcinoma, which occurs in about 5 percent of all infected patients.[16]

Currently, three interferons, IFN-α 2a, IFN-α 2b, and IFN-α con-1, are approved for the treatment of chronic HCV.

Multiple myeloma. Multiple myeloma is a B-lymphocyte malignancy in which high levels of monoclonal antibodies are produced. The transformed B-lymphocyte requires high levels of interleukin-6 to sustain its proliferation and survival. It was recently found that patients with multiple myeloma were infected with HHV-8 in bone marrow stroma cells. The HHV-8-infected stroma cells produce a cytokine that is a homolog of IL-6, which is able to induce proliferation of these transformed B-cells.[16]

The primary treatment of multiple myeloma is cytotoxic chemotherapy consisting of cyclophosphamide, doxorubicin, and dexamethasone (CAD). Although effective in producing remission of disease, CAD is unable to produce a durable response. In this scenario, IFN-α has been used. rhIFN-α is able to modulate both paracrine and autocrinic IL-6 expression. Other immunomodulator activities include activation of NK cells and CTLs that eliminate cancerous cells. One method to increase immunological response against myeloma is rhIFN-α-induced expression of MHC class I in tumor cells. This will allow the effector cells to recognize and exert cytotoxic effects on malignant cells. Doses of IFN-α in the treatment of multiple myeloma range from 3 to 5 MU given daily as a SC or IM injection.[16]

Acute T-cell leukemia/lymphoma. Acute T-cell leukemia/lymphoma (ATL) and mycosis fungoides are hematological conditions that have been associated with human T-cell leukemia virus I (HTLV-I) infections. The clinical presentation includes (1) hypercalcemia, (2) elevated PTH, (3) elevated CD4+ cells, (4) CD4+ cells acting as suppresser T-cells, and (5) elevated IL-10 levels.[16]

HTLV-I is a retrovirus that can be transmitted through intimate contact similar to HIV and the hepatitis viruses. When infected cells are transformed, causing the development of leukemia or lymphoma, high levels of interleukin-10 (IL-10) expression (a cytokine that has T-cell inhibitory activity and suppresses the expansion of CTLs and NK cells) occurs. In addition, IL-10 can up-regulate interleukin-1 receptor antagonist (IL-1ra), a naturally occurring antagonist that competes for receptor binding without any stimulatory activity. The expression of IL-10 and IL-1ra will down-regulate the immune response, which may explain why patients with ATL have suppressed cellular immunity and are susceptible to opportunistic infections, such as *Pneumocystis carinii* pneumonia (PCP).[16]

Presently, there is no effective chemotherapeutic treatment for HTLV-I associated ATL, and five-year survival is less than 10 percent. However, progression of disease can be inhibited by using antiviral therapy such as the combination of IFN-α and dideoxynucleoside analogs such as zidovudine (AZT). When 5 MU of IFN-α is combined with 300 mg of AZT three times daily, complete remission from ATL has been realized. This is a durable response when the disappearance of HTLV-I is associated with prolonged remission.[22]

Adverse Reactions

Adverse effects associated with IFN-α therapy are summarized in Box 5.2. All patients receiving interferon-α develop flulike symptoms in a dose-dependent manner.[19,20,21] This observance has been attributed to the induction of proinflammatory cytokines such as IL-1 and TNF.

Interferon-β

As previously mentioned, interferon-β (IFN-β) binds onto Type I IFN receptor, explaining its similar biological activity to IFN-α. Presently, there are two commercially available IFN-β products, named IFN-β 1a (Avenox) and IFN-β 1b (Betaseron), as reviewed in Table 5.7. These products gained FDA approval for the treatment of multiple sclerosis (MS), a neurological disorder characterized by a loss in motor function.

BOX 5.2. Adverse Reactions of Interferon-α

- Flulike syndromes
  ⇒ Chills
  ⇒ Fever
- Musculoskeletal effects
  ⇒ Myalgias
  ⇒ Arthralgias
- Gastrointestinal effects
  ⇒ Gastrointestinal upset
- Thyroid dysfunction
  ⇒ Drop in T3 and T4
- Hematological effects
  ⇒ Neutropenia
  ⇒ Anemia
- Hepatic effects
  ⇒ Elevated liver enzymes
  ⇒ Elevated transaminases
  ⇒ Elevated alkaline phosphatase

TABLE 5.7. Comparison of Interferon-β 1a and 1b

	Interferon-β 1a	Interferon-β 1b
Trade name	Avenox	Betaserone
Expression cell	Chinese hamster ovary cell	*Escherichia coli*
Number of amino acids	166	165
Molecular weight	22.5 kDa	18.5 kDa
Carbohydrate side chains	Yes	No
Activity	200 MU/mg	32 MU/mg
Vial size	0.03 mg/vial	0.3 mg/vial
Albumin	15 mg/vial	15 mg/vial

IFN-β exerts its anti-MS activity via down-regulation of T-cell activation. This is accomplished through down modulating IFN-γ, TNF-α, and lymphotoxin (TNF-β) protein expression. Patients who are receiving IFN-β were found to produce high levels of transforming growth factor β (TGF-β), a cytokine with immunosuppressive activity. Although IFN-β has antitumor activity, its antineoplastic activity is still not fully understood. The administration of IFN-β has been an effective treatment against gliomas, breast cancer, and bladder cancer.

Similar to other IFNs, IFN-β has been shown to possess both antiviral and immunomodulatory activities. The exact mechanism by which IFN-β 1a and 1b exert their biological activities is not clearly defined. Biological activities require that IFN-β bind onto Type I IFN receptors, which stimulate transcription of various genes known as IFN-stimulated genes (ISG). The transcription of 2',5'-oligoadenylate synthetase, protein kinase, and indoleamine 2,3-dioxygenase are believed to be the mediators of IFN-β biological activity.[16]

Interferon-β 1a, Recombinant (Avenox®)

Product information. Interferon-β 1a (INF-β 1a) is indicated for use in patients with relapsing forms of multiple sclerosis. It is stated to slow the accumulation of physical disability and decrease the frequency of clinical exacerbations.

IFN-β 1a is produced by insertion of the native IFN-β gene. Unlike IFN-β 1b, the modified plasmid containing the IFN-β 1a gene is introduced into a chinese hamster ovary (CHO) expression system. The purified recombinant product is a glycoprotein consisting of 166 amino acids. The molecular weight IFN-β 1a is 22.5 kDa, which is substantially larger than IFN-β 1b. Glycosylation not only increases the molecular weight but is an important factor determining biological activity. This is demonstrated by IFN-β 1a having a specific activity of 200 MU/mg versus only 32 MU/mg for the unglycosylated IFN-β 1b product.[23]

Clinical trials—Multiple sclerosis. The clinical effects of IFN-β 1a in multiple sclerosis were studied in a randomized, multicenter, double-blind, placebo-controlled study in patients with relapsing (stable or progressive) MS. In this study, 301 patients received either 6 million IU (30 μg) of IFN-β 1a (*n*=158) or placebo (*n*=143) by IM injection once weekly. Patients received IFN-β 1a injections for up to two years, and continued to be followed until study completion. There were 144 patients treated with IFN-β 1a for more than one year; 115 patients were able to complete 18 months, and 82 patients completed two years of therapy.

All patients had a definite diagnosis of MS of at least one year in duration, and had at least two exacerbations in the three years prior to study entry (or one per year if the duration of disease was less than three years). At study entry, patients had to be free of exacerbation during the prior two months and Kurtzke Expanded Disability Status Scale (EDSS) scores had to range from 1.0 to 3.5. All patients with chronic progressive MS were excluded from this study. The primary outcome assessment was time to progression in disability. This was measured as an increase in EDSS score of at least 1.0 point, sustained for at least six months. Secondary outcomes included the frequency of exacerbation and gadolinium (Gd)-enhancing lesions on MRI scans.

IFN-β 1a was able to significantly delay time to onset of disability as compared to patients treated with placebo (p value = 0.02). Kaplan-Meier estimation suggested that patients receiving placebo had a 34.9 percent chance of increased disability, whereas patients treated with IFN-β 1a had a 21.9 percent chance of disease progression for the same period. This represented a 37 percent reduction in the risk of accumulating disability.[23]

IFN-β 1a treatment significantly decreased the frequency of exacerbation in the subset of patients who were enrolled in the study for at least two years (87 placebo-treated patients and 85 IFN-β 1a-treated patients; p value = 0.03). The annual MS exacerbation rate was 0.67 per year in the IFN-β 1a-treated group, and 0.82 per year in the placebo-treated group (p value = 0.04).

Secondary end points such as Gd enhancements and T2-weighted (proton density) magnetic resonance imaging (MRI) scans of the brain were obtained in most patients at baseline and at the end of one and two years of treatment. Gd-enhancing lesions seen on brain MRI scans represent areas of blood-brain barrier breakdown thought to be secondary to inflammation. Patients treated with IFN-β 1a demonstrated significantly lower Gd-enhanced lesion numbers after one and two years of treatment (p value ≤ 0.05). The volume of Gd-enhanced lesions was also analyzed and showed similar treatment effects (p value ≤ 0.03). The percentage change in T2-weighted lesion volume from study entry to year one was significantly lower in IFN-β 1a-treated as compared to placebo-treated patients (p value = 0.02). However, statistical significance was not observed at the end of two years.

Adverse reactions. The safety of IFN-β 1a in MS patients is based on a placebo-controlled trial in which 158 patients were treated for up to two years. The most common adverse events associated with IFN-β 1a treatment were flulike symptoms including myalgias, arthralgias, fever, chills, and asthenia. However, the incidence of flulike events diminished with continued treatment. Subcutaneous injections were also associated with the following local reactions at injection site: necrosis, atrophy, edema, and hemorrhage.[23]

Neurological events, such as depression and seizures, were notable. Although depression occurred in patients randomized to receive IFN-β 1a, the incidence of depression was equal in the two treatment groups. Since suicidal ideation has been reported with other interferon products, IFN-β 1a should be used with caution. Four patients receiving IFN-β 1a experienced seizures, whereas no seizures were reported in the placebo group. History of seizures were absent in 3 out of 4 patients; however, it is not known whether these events were related to the effects of MS, IFN-β 1a therapy, or a combination of the two.

Interferon-β 1b, Recombinant (Betaseron®)

Product information. Interferon-β 1b (IFN-β 1b or Betaseron) is approved for the treatment of relapsing multiple sclerosis. Using recombinant DNA technology, the native IFN-β gene was isolated from human fibroblasts, which was modified by replacing a serine for cysteine residue at the seventeenth position. The recombinant plasmid was inserted into an *E. coli* expression system to produce an unglycosylated recombinant product. The purified IFN-β 1b product consists of 165 amino acids in its polypeptide backbone with a molecular weight of 18.9 kDa.[24]

Pharmacokinetics. The pharmacokinetic parameters of IFN-β are reviewed in Table 5.8. These parameters were not derived from patients with MS, rather they were reported from healthy male patients. One notable difference between the two products is the bioavailability after a subcutaneous dose. IFN-β 1a has a bioavailability of 16.6 percent while IFN-β 1b has a bioavailability of 50 percent after a subcutaneous dose.

Other pharmacokinetics parameters are relatively similar between the two IFN-β products, suggesting glycosylation has relatively little to do with pharmacokinetics. Following a single subcutaneous dose of IFN-β 1a, the half-life was five hours, whereas the half-life of IFN-β 1b was 4.3 hours. Other parameters such as maximum achieved concentration (Cmax) were similar between the two products; 45 and 40 IU/mL were achieved using either IFN-β 1a or IFN-β 1b. Both have similar clearance profiles; the rate of elimination for IFN-β 1a

TABLE 5.8. Pharmacokinetic Parameters of Interferon-β 1

Parameters	Interferon-β 1a	Interferon-β 1b
Bioavailability	16.6% percent SC	50% percent SC
AUC (IU/h per mL)	1,353 (IM) 478 (SC)	NA
Half-life	10 h ($t_{1/2\beta}$)	4.3 h ($t_{1/2\beta}$)
Tmax (Range)	7.8 h (3-18 h) SC	1-8 h SC
Cmax (IU/mL)	45 (IM)	40 (SC)
Volume of Distribution	NA	0.25-2.88 L/kg
Clearance	100 L/h (1.4 L/h per kg)	9.4-28.9 mL/min per kg (0.564 to 1.734 L/h per kg)

was 100 L/h (1.4 L/h per kg), and IFN-β 1b exhibited a range from 0.564 to 1.734 L/h per kg.[23]

Biologic pharmacodynamic effects persisted even when IFN-β 1a serum levels had returned to baseline and were still significantly elevated three days after a single dose. Extent and duration of clinical and biologic effects were independent of the route of administration and of the IFN-β 1a serum levels. The SC route of administration is preferred for instances in which an immunomodulatory action is primarily sought. Predominantly, antiviral and antiproliferative activity is enhanced by the intravenous route providing adequate drug levels at the site of pathology. However, practical application is still limited.

Low levels of free IFN-β 1b are difficult to detect following subcutaneous administration of 0.25 mg. Following a single injection of 0.5 mg of IFN-β 1b, serum levels were generally below 100 IU/mL. Peak concentration was achieved in one to eight hours with a mean serum peak of 40 IU/mL.[23]

Clinical trials—Multiple sclerosis. The effectiveness of IFN-β 1b was evaluated in 372 ambulatory patients with relapsing MS. All patients had Poser's criteria 13 for clinically definite and/or laboratory supported diagnosis of MS. In addition, patients had to have a history of at least two exacerbations over the last two years, in which the last episode occurred more than one month prior to enrollment. All patients must have never used any immunosuppressive agents such as steroids and azathioprine.

Patients were randomized into one of three groups: placebo (*n* = 123), 0.05 mg of IFN-β 1b, or 0.25 mg (*n* = 124) in which patients self-administered IFN-β subcutaneously every other day. In this two-year trial, clinical end points were (1) frequency of MS exacerbation per patient and (2) proportion of patients who were free of MS exacerbation. A number of secondary outcome measures were also determined. A substudy of patients was assessed using annual magnetic resonance imaging. MRIs were used to quantify the extent of disease as determined by changes in total area of lesions. More intensive MRI studies were performed at one site (*n* = 52), where imaging studies were performed every six weeks.

After two years of treatment, withdrawal from study varied with treatment assignment. Excessive use of steroids accounted for 11 of the 26 withdrawals from the placebo group, whereas only 2 out of 21 patients withdrew from the study due to excessive steroids in patients who were receiving 0.05 mg, and 1 out of 25 withdrew in the group receiving 0.25 mg. Withdrawals attributed to adverse events were more common among IFN-β 1b-treated patients: one, five, and ten withdrew from the placebo, 0.05 mg, and 0.25 mg groups, respectively.

In the two-year analysis, there was a 31 percent reduction in annual exacerbation rate, from 1.31 in the placebo group to 0.9 in the group receiving 0.25 mg of IFN-β 1b (p value = 0.0001). The proportion of patients free of exacerbation was 16 percent in the placebo group, as compared to 25 percent in the (IFN-β 1b) 0.25 mg group.

Over the two-year period, there were 25 MS-related hospitalizations in patients who were receiving 0.25 mg IFN-β 1b as compared to 48 hospitalizations in the placebo group. In comparison, non-MS hospitalizations were evenly distributed among the groups, with 16 in the 0.25 mg IFN-β 1b group, while 15 patients required non-MS-related hospitalization in the placebo group. Average days of MS-related steroid use were 41 in the 0.25 mg IFN-β 1b group and 55 in the placebo group (p value = 0.004).

MRI scanning is viewed as a useful means to visualize changes in white matter which are believed to be a reflection of the pathologic changes that, appropriately located within the central nervous system (CNS), account for some of the signs and symptoms that typify relapsing-remitting MS. Analysis of MRI data suggested a significant lesion reduction was observed in patients receiving 0.25 mg of IFN-β 1b as compared to placebo, whereas patients receiving the drug had 1.1 percent of lesion expansion as compared to 16.5 percent in patients receiving placebo (p value = 0.0001). When more intensive MRI studies were performed (every six weeks), new or expanding lesions were found in 29 percent of patients receiving placebo, while only 6 percent patients had new or expanding lesions in the 0.25 mg treatment group (p value = 0.006).

As noted, in the two-year analysis, there was a 31 percent reduction in exacerbation rate in the 0.25 mg group, compared with placebo. The p value for this difference was 0.0001. In the analysis of the third year alone, the difference between treatment groups was 28 percent. The p value was 0.065. The lower number of patients may account for the loss of statistical significance; lack of direct comparability among the patient groups in this extension study makes the interpretation of these results difficult.

Throughout the clinical trial, serum samples from the patients were monitored for the development of antibodies to IFN-β 1b; 45 percent of the patients on 0.25 mg of IFN-β 1b (n = 124) developed neutralizing activity.[23]

Adverse reactions. IFN-β 1b is well tolerated with only mild to moderate adverse events. The only severe adverse events reported were inflammation, pain, and necrosis. Injection site reaction was the most frequently encountered event, which occurred in about 79 percent of patients during the first three months of treatment. Incidence of injection reaction reduced to 47 percent during the last six months.[23]

Flulike symptoms occurred in 76 percent of patients who received IFN-β 1b. Flulike symptoms were defined as symptoms that included fevers, chills, myalgias, malaise, or sweating, which were similar to injection reactions as the frequency decreased with time.

The incidence for flulike symptom complex was also calculated over the course of three years. The incidence rate of flulike symptoms decreased over time, where 60 percent of patients experienced these types of events during the first three months. This was substantially lower (down to 10 percent) during the last six months of therapy. The median time to the first occurrence of flulike symptom complex was 3.5 days, where the median duration per patient was 7.5 days per year.

Laboratory abnormalities included absolute neutrophil count less than 1,500/mm³ (18 percent) (no patients had absolute neutrophil counts less than 500/mm³), WBC (white blood cell) count less than 3,000/mm³ (16 percent), alanine aminotransferase (SGPT) greater than five times baseline value (19 percent), and total bilirubin greater than 2.5 times baseline value (6 percent). Three patients were withdrawn from treatment with 0.25 mg IFN-β 1b for abnormal liver enzymes, including one following dose reduction.[23]

Twenty-one (28 percent) of the 76 premenopausal females treated at 0.25 mg IFN-β 1b and ten (13 percent) of the 76 premenopausal females treated with placebo reported menstrual disorders. All of these reports were of mild to moderate severity and included intermenstrual bleeding and spotting, early or delayed menses, decreased days of menstrual flow, and clotting and spotting during menstruation. Mental disorders have been observed in patients in this study. Symptoms included depression, anxiety, emotional lability, depersonalization, suicide attempts, and confusion, etc. In the treatment group, two patients withdrew due to experiencing confusion. One suicide and four attempted suicides were also reported. It is not known whether these symptoms were related to the underlying neurological basis of MS, to IFN-β 1b treatment, or to a combination of both factors. Some similar symptoms that have been noted in patients receiving IFN-α 1a are thought to act through the same receptor. Patients who experienced these types of symptoms should be closely monitored and cessation therapy should be considered.

Interferon-γ

Naturally occurring interferon-γ 1a (IFN-γ) binds onto the Type II IFN receptor. This glycoprotein has a 143 amino acid polypeptide backbone with a molecular weight of 20 to 25 kDa, which is dependent on the degree of glycosylation. Naturally occurring IFN-γ is produced primarily by activated T-lymphocytes and natural killer cells.

The biological activity of IFN-γ includes the activation of phagocytic activities of resting monocytes and macrophages. Cells that have been treated with IFN-γ will have increased production of reactive oxygen radicals, which will exert its antimicrobial activity. In addition, IFN-γ can enhance antibody-dependent cellular-mediated cytotoxicity (ADCC). As with any IFN, IFN-γ has antiviral activity. However, its antiviral activity is less when compared to other IFNs such as IFN-α.

Interferon-γ 1b, Recombinant (Actimmune®)

Product information. Recombinant human IFN-γ 1b (rhIFN-γ 1b or Actimmune) is a single-chain polypeptide, with 140 amino acids, that was expressed in *E. coli*. rhIFN-γ 1b has a molecular weight of 16.5 kDa, with a specific biological activity of 30 MU/mg. Presently, rhIFN-γ 1b is approved for use in patients with chronic granulomatous disease (CGD), an autoimmune disease that affects the lungs.[25] Patients afflicted with CGD have a lower capacity to perform phagocytic oxidative metabolism. When these patients are given recombinant human IFN-γ, normal production of reactive oxygen radicals is correlated with an increased capacity for phagocytic oxidative metabolism. When these patients are given recombinant human IFN-γ

1b, normal production of reactive oxygen radicals is demonstrated. Increased formation of reactive oxygen radicals is correlated with an increased capacity to phagocytize *Staphylococcus aureus* and eliminate bacteria.[16]

Pharmacokinetics. The pharmacokinetics of IFN-γ 1b have not been investigated in patients with chronic granulomatous disease. Instead, the pharmacokinetic parameters have been characterized in healthy male subjects (Table 5.9). IFN-γ 1b is slowly absorbed after intramuscular and subcutaneous injection, where the bioavailability is greater than 89 percent. The elimination half-life after IV administration of 100 μg/m² was 38 minutes, whereas a longer half-life was seen when it was administered via IM (2.9 hours) or SC (5.9 hours) routes. After an IV dose of IFN-γ 1b, the clearance was reported to be 1.4 L/min. Time to peak concentrations occurred four hours and seven hours after an IM or SC dose of 100 μg/m², where the concentrations were 1.5 ng/mL and 0.6 ng/mL, respectively.[25]

The intravenous, intramuscular, and subcutaneous pharmacokinetics of IFN-γ 1b were investigated in 24 healthy male subjects following single-dose administration of 100 μg/m². IFN-γ 1b is rapidly cleared after intravenous administration (1.4 L/min) and slowly absorbed after intramuscular or subcutaneous injection. After intramuscular or subcutaneous injection, the apparent fraction of dose absorbed was greater than 89 percent. The mean elimination half-life after intravenous administration of 100 μg/m² in healthy male subjects was 38 minutes. The mean elimination half-lives for intramuscular and subcutaneous dosing with 100 μg/m² were 2.9 and 5.9 hours, respectively. Peak plasma concentrations, determined by ELISA (enzyme-linked immunosorbent assay), occurred approximately four hours (1.5 ng/mL) after intramuscular dosing and seven hours (0.6 ng/mL) after subcu-

TABLE 5.9. Pharmacokinetics of Interferon-γ 1b

Pharmacokinetic Parameter	Value
Absorption	89 percent (IM or SC)
Tmax	4 h (IM), 7 h (SC)
Cmax	1.5 ng/mL (IM), 0.6 ng/mL (SC)
Clearance	1.4 L/min
Half-life	38 min (IV), 2.9 h (IM), 5.9 h (SC)

taneous dosing. Multiple-dose subcutaneous pharmacokinetic studies were conducted in 38 healthy male subjects. There was no accumulation of IFN-γ 1b after 12 consecutive daily injections of 100 μg/m^2.

Excretion studies of IFN-γ 1b have been performed. Trace amounts of interferon-γ were detected in the urine of squirrel monkeys following intravenous administration of 500 μg/kg. IFN-γ 1b was not detected in the urine of healthy human volunteers following administration of 100 μg/m^2 of IFN-γ 1b by the intravenous, intramuscular, and subcutaneous routes. In vitro perfusion studies utilizing rabbit livers and kidneys demonstrate that these organs are capable of clearing interferon-γ from perfusate. Studies of the administration of interferon-γ to nephrectomized mice and squirrel monkeys demonstrate a reduction in its clearance from blood; however, prior nephrectomy did not prevent elimination.

Clinical trials—Chronic granulomatous disease. Chronic granulomatous disease (CGD) is a rare X-linked or autosomal genetic disorder affecting phagocytes in the host defense. More specifically, individuals with CGD have a defect in the NADPH oxidase system which is important in host defense against various microorganisms (Table 5.10). The resultant effect is decreased production of superoxide radicals, which is an important component of microbicidal mechanism. A reduction of superoxide formation can lead to recurrent, serious, life-threatening infections and granuloma formation. The most commonly encountered recurrent infections are catalase-positive microorganisms such as *Staphylococcus aureus* and *Aspergillus* species. Other organisms that are frequently encountered in CGD patients include *Serratia marcescens, Pseudomonas cepacia, Escherichia coli, Klebsiella,* and *Nocardia* species.[16]

TABLE 5.10. Types of Chronic Granulomatous Diseases

Genetic Trait	Frequency	Defect
X-linked	60%	91 kDa component of membrane-bound oxidase
Autosomal recessive	30%	47 kDa cystolic protein
Autosomal recessive	<5%	22 kDa component of cytochrome b-558
Autosomal recessive	<5%	65 kDa cytosolic protein
Autosomal dominant	<1%	47 kDa protein

CGD is a heterogeneous disorder that is characterized by a disorder of phagocytic oxidative metabolism. CGD can occur as a result of defects in either the cytosolic or membrane component of the NADPH oxidase system. Estimates suggest that 60 percent of patients have a defect in the membrane oxidase system which involves the 91 kDa component of cytochrome b-558, whereas individuals with cytosolic defects are linked to patients with autosomal recessive traits. The majority of these patients have a defect in 47 kDa cytosolic protein of the cytochrome b-558 complex.

The clinical symptoms associated with CGD were found to be ameliorated when patients afflicted with this disorder were given IFN-γ 1b. The addition can potentiate phagocyte activity thus restoring some defective phagocyte NADPH oxidase system activity.[16]

In a clinical large-scale study of the efficacy of IFN-γ 1b in comparison with placebo, patients receiving IFN-γ 1b had a significant reduction in the incidence of serious clinical events necessitating hospitalization. This translated into a decreased risk of developing serious infection, thus leading to a decrease in the number of patients needing hospitalization. Patients receiving IFN-γ 1b had a reduced incidence of clinical events that required hospitalization by 67 percent as compared to those receiving placebo. In addition, the group receiving IFN-γ 1b had a twofold reduction in the number of serious infections, which was defined as infections requiring parenteral antibiotics and hospitalization. This translated to a dramatic drop in hospitalization; patients in the placebo group had 56 events as compared to 20 (p value < 0.0001). The number of days in the hospital was 1,493 versus 497 between the two groups, respectively. Furthermore, hospital stay was necessary in about one-third of patients who developed infection.

All patients receiving the drug had improved clinical outcomes regardless of age, sex, use of prophylactic antibiotics, or genetic pattern of inheritance. However, IFN-γ 1b provided the greatest therapeutic benefit to patients who were less than ten years of age.

Adverse reactions. IFN-γ 1b is well tolerated with the most common adverse effects listed in Table 5.11. Effects are usually mild, transient, and relieved by symptomatic treatment. IFN-γ 1b, therefore, provides an effective and well-tolerated therapy for patients with chronic granulomatous disease, offering an important clinical

TABLE 5.11. Adverse Effect Profile of Interferon-γ 1b

Clinical Toxicity	IFN-γ 1b (%)	Placebo (%)
Fever	52	28
Headache	33	9
Rash	17	6
Chills	14	0
Injection site erythema or tenderness	14	2
Fatigue	14	11
Diarrhea	14	12
Vomiting	13	5
Nausea	10	2
Weight loss	6	6
Myalgias	6	0
Anorexia	3	5
Arthralgia	2	0
Injection site pain	0	2

advance in the treatment of this rare genetic disorder by improving the prognosis of its serious and life-threatening infectious sequelae.

The most common adverse experiences occurring with IFN-γ 1b therapy are flulike or constitutional symptoms such as fever, headache, chills, myalgias, or fatigue, which may decrease in severity as treatment continues. Some of the flulike symptoms may be minimized by bedtime administration. Acetaminophen may be used to prevent or partially alleviate the fever and headache. The long-term effects of IFN-γ 1b therapy on growth, development, or other parameters are not known. In addition to those tests normally required for monitoring patients with CGD, complete blood counts and renal and liver function tests should be performed on all patients receiving IFN-γ 1b therapy prior to the beginning of and at three-month intervals during treatment.[25]

The data on adverse reactions are based on the subcutaneous administration of IFN-γ 1b at a dose of 50 μg/m², three times weekly, in 63 patients with CGD during an investigational trial in the United States and Europe. Sixty-five additional patients with CGD received placebo in this study.

COLONY-STIMULATING FACTORS

Hematopoietic Growth Factors

Colony-stimulating factors (CSFs) are hematopoietic growth factors (HGFs) that regulate the commitment, proliferation, maturation, and function of myeloid cells (Figure 5.3). HGFs are glycoproteins that are primarily produced by either stimulated T-lymphocytes or macrophages. In various inflammatory events, endothelial cells and fibroblasts have also been known to produce CSFs. CSFs act on

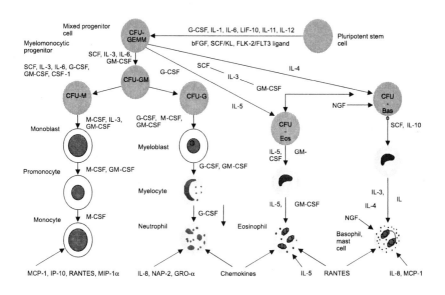

FIGURE 5.3. Hematopoietic growth factors in myeloid maturation (*Source:* Adapted from Abboud and Liesveld. In Hoffman R, Benz EJ Jr., Shattil SJ, Furie B, Cohen HJ, Siberstein LE, McGlave P. (Eds.), *Hematology: Basic principles and practice,* Third edition. 2000:223.)

hematopoietic cells by binding onto their specific membrane receptors, thus stimulating proliferation, differentiation, commitment, and functional activation.

Despite their overlapping biological activities, each CSF has its own distinctive structure, with little structural homology between the CSFs. CSFs are organized as either Class I or II CSFs, where Class I CSFs have multilineage activities. In contrast, Class II CSFs, or unipotent CSFs, have biological activity that is restricted to only one type of circulating cell. In addition, Class II CSFs exert their biological activities when hematopoietic cells are more mature in nature.[16]

Myeloid growth factors, such as granulocyte-macrophage colony-stimulating factors and multilineage CSF (Multi-CSF), or interleukin-3 (IL-3), are classified as pluripotent or Class I CSFs, whereas granulocyte CSF (G-CSF), macrophage CSF (M-CSF), erythropoietin (EPO), thrombopoietin (TPO), and megakaryocyte-derived growth factor (MDGF) are all members of unipotent or Class II CSFs. These factors work in concert to form mature and functional circulating cells from the totipotent hematopoietic stem cell.

Human Granulocyte Colony-Stimulating Factor

Natural or endogenous granulocyte colony-stimulating factor (G-CSF) is a lineage specific CSF, which is produced primarily by monocytes, fibroblasts, and endothelial cells. G-CSF regulates the production of neutrophils and neutrophil progenitor proliferation, as well as differentiation. The binding of G-CSF onto the G-CSF receptor will result in activation of neutrophil functions which include enhanced phagocytic ability, respiratory burst, antibody-dependent killing, and expression of some functions associated with cell surface antigens.[16]

Humans who have undetectable levels of the G-CSF usually have chronic neutropenia. The neutrophils isolated from these patients are unable to mobilize to the affected sites. It is therefore understandable that these individuals are very susceptible to bacterial infections.

When G-CSF was administered to animals, significant toxicities were not apparent in mice, rats, hamsters, or monkeys. No deaths associated with G-CSF were reported in these animal studies. In dose-tolerance studies, evidence of neurological symptoms was seen in monkeys treated with doses of recombinant G-CSF greater than

1,150 µg/kg per day for up to 18 days. In a study that lasted 52 weeks, one female monkey died after 18 weeks of daily IV doses of 115 µg/kg per day. Death was attributed to cardiopulmonary insufficiency. In all species, histopathologic examination of the liver and spleen revealed evidence of progressive extramedullary granulopoiesis, which resulted in dose-dependent increased spleen weights. In general, adverse effects developed in a dose-dependent manner, where increase in serum alkaline phosphatase was observed. The activities of osteoblasts and osteoclasts were significantly increased, where laboratory values were reversible following discontinuation of treatment.

Filgrastim (Neupogen®)

Product information. Filgrastim or recombinant human G-CSF (rhG-CSF) is indicated to reduce the incidence of infection in patients with nonmyeloid malignancies and febrile neutropenia. It is also indicated for use in the treatment of acute myeloid leukemia. This product is produced by insertion of human G-CSF gene into an *E. coli* expression system. The G-CSF gene has been altered such that a N-terminal methionine is absent in the recombinant product. rhG-CSF is nonglycosylated with biological activity identical to the naturally occurring agent.[21]

Pharmacokinetics. The pharmacokinetic parameters of rhG-CSF are reviewed in Table 5.12. After the administration of rhG-CSF, this recombinant product follows a first-order pharmacokinetic profile which is not concentration dependent. When rhG-CSF was administered as a continuous IV infusion (20 µg/kg) over 24 hours, mean and

TABLE 5.12. Pharmacokinetics of rhG-CSF

Pharmacokinetic Parameter	Value
Cmax	4-49 ng/mL (3.45-11.5 µcg/kg SC)
	384 ng/mL (11.5 µcg/kg IV over 3 min)
Cl	0.5-0.7 mL/min per kg
$t_{1/2}$	3.5 h
Vd	150 mL per kg
Absorption clearance	0.5-0.7 mL/min per kg

median serum concentrations of approximately 48 and 56 ng/mL, respectively, were measured.[26] However, when administered as subcutaneous injections (3.45 µg/kg and 11.5 µg/kg), maximum serum concentrations (Cmax) was measured at 4 and 49 ng/mL, respectively. The distribution of rhG-CSF was similar in both normal subjects and cancer patients where the average volume distribution (Vd) was 150 mL/kg. The elimination half-life, in both normal subjects and cancer patients, was approximately 3.5 hours, whereas the rate of elimination for rhG-CSF was measured to be 0.5 to 0.7 mL/min per kg. Single parenteral doses or daily IV doses, over a 14-day period, resulted in comparable half-lives. Continuous 24-hour IV infusions of 20 µg/kg over an 11- to 20-day period produced steady-state serum concentrations of rhG-CSF with no evidence of drug accumulation over the time period investigated.[26]

Clinical trials in prevention of chemotherapy-induced neutropenia. One major drawback to cancer cytotoxic chemotherapy agents is that they are unable to discriminate between tumor and self cells. This inability to selectively kill tumor cells can lead to adverse events, such as alopecia, nausea, vomiting, diarrhea, mucositis, and myelosuppression. Common hematological toxicities can manifest anemia, thrombocytopenia, and neutropenia. The major sequelae in severe neutropenic patients increase the risk of developing life-threatening infections.[16]

Since neutrophil plays a critical role in the defense against microbial invaders, it is not surprising that patients with neutropenia are susceptible to bacterial infections. In particular, neutropenic patients seem to be susceptible to enteric gram-negative bacteria that enter the circulation through the gastrointestinal tract. The combination of myelosuppression and increased transit of bacteria into circulation will increase the risk of life-threatening infections.

To assess the effects of rhG-CSF, 96 patients with various non-myeloid malignancies were given rhG-CSF. The administration of rhG-CSF resulted in a dose-dependent increase in circulating neutrophil counts over the dosage range of 1 to 70 µg/kg per day. An increase in absolute neutrophil counts (ANCs) was observed regardless of parenteral route of administration. rhG-CSF directly affected the level of circulating neutrophils. This was most evident when ANC dropped after the discontinuation of rhG-CSF. In most patients, ANC returned to baseline levels within four days after the discontinuation of rhG-CSF therapy.[26]

Although absolute monocyte count also increased in a dose-dependent manner, monocytes remained in the normal range throughout drug administration. As expected, the number of eosinophils and basophils did not change during rhG-CSF administration. Furthermore, lymphocyte counts were unaltered by the presence of neutrophil factor. White blood cell differentials obtained during clinical trials have demonstrated a shift toward earlier granulocyte progenitor cells (left shift), including the appearance of neutrophil precursors such as promyelocytes and myeloblasts.

The safety of rhG-CSF was evaluated in patients with transitional cell carcinoma (TCCA) receiving cytotoxic chemotherapy. During cycles in which rhG-CSF was given, patients' neutrophil counts recovered rapidly, which allowed all the patients to receive their scheduled chemotherapy. During cycles in which rhG-CSF support was withdrawn, only 33 percent of the patients were able to receive their scheduled chemotherapy on time as measured by ANCs and WBC counts.

In the phase III pivotal trial, rhG-CSF was evaluated on its ability to prevent infections in small-cell lung carcinoma (SCLC) patients who were to receive a chemotherapy regimen consisting of cyclophosphamide, doxorubicin, and etoposide (CAE). These patients were randomized in a double-blinded fashion to receive either rhG-CSF or diluent (placebo). Patients who were randomized to receive rhG-CSF had significantly shorter duration of severe neutropenia than those receiving placebo. rhG-CSF-induced recovery of circulating neutrophils were able to prevent the development of neutropenic fevers that are common in cancer patients receiving chemotherapy. A drop in neutropenic fevers translated to a 47 percent reduction of antibiotic usage, which corresponded to a reduction in hospitalization associated with neutropenia.[26]

Clinical trials with G-CSF in HIV. A hallmark of patients with HIV is global decline in circulating cells. This is attributed to the reduction of CD4+ cells which regulate stimulatory cytokine expression. In an effort to stimulate the immune system, stimulatory cytokines, such as GM-CSF and G-CSF, have been employed.

The administration of rhG-CSF was able to increase the number of neutrophils in patients with HIV. Neutrophils isolated from HIV patients treated with rhG-CSF showed enhanced neutrophil functions, even in patients previously diagnosed with neutrophil dysfunction. Increased microcidal activities were evident from the increased neutrophil-myeloperoxidase and chemotactic activity.

Less rhG-CSF was required in the HIV patients to give the same level of WBC elevation as in cancer patients. The effect of rhG-CSF and epoietin alfa were evaluated in patients with either AIDS or AIDS-related complex (ARC) who had antiviral-agent-induced anemia and leukopenia. These patients had a four-week washout period where all myelosuppressive agents were discontinued. Patients were initially given 1.2 µg/kg per day rhG-CSF, which showed a significant ANC increase (p value < 0.05). After reaching targeted ANC, patients were started on 150 units/kg of epoeitin alfa, given three times a week. All patients were able to achieve or surpass the target hemoglobin levels within five weeks of therapy. In the fourth stage of this study, patients were reinitiated on zidovudine at 1,000 to 1,500 mg/day given orally in five divided doses. A dose increase ranging from 0.3 to 1.2 µg/kg per day of rhG-CSF was required to maintain the target ANC in these patients. This study suggests that two cytokines could be coadministered without affecting other hematological indices.

Adverse reactions. The adverse effect profile documented the experience of 207 patients. In this study, no serious, life-threatening, or fatal adverse reactions were attributed to filgrastim therapy. Unlike rhGM-CSF, no reports of flulike symptoms, pleuritis, pericarditis, or other major systemic reactions was attributed to rhG-CSF.[26]

Adverse effects experienced by patients included reversible elevations in uric acid, lactate dehydrogenase, and alkaline phosphatase, which occurred in 27 to 58 percent in patients who received rhG-CSF. Although 7 out of 176 patients experienced transient decreases in blood pressure ($< 90/60$ mmHg), no clinical treatment was required. In addition, cardiac events, such as myocardial infarctions and arrhythmias, occurred in 11 of 375 cancer patients; however, the relationship to rhG-CSF therapy has not been ascertained.[26]

Granulocyte Macrophage Colony-Stimulating Factor

Granulocyte macrophage colony-stimulating factor (GM-CSF) is a pluripotent myeloid growth factor that supports survival, clonal expansion, and differentiation of hematopoietic progenitor cells in a concentration-dependent manner.[1] In its natural form, GM-CSF is able to support the differentiation of granulocytes and macrophage precursors. In vitro studies have demonstrated that GM-CSF can promote proliferation of other myeloid precursors, such as megakaryocytic, erythroid progenitor cells, in a dose-dependent manner. In addition, GM-CSF was able to increase monocyte chemotaxis against fungus and parasites.

Sargramostim, GM-CSF (Leukine®)

Product information. Recombinant human GM-CSF (rhGM-CSF) or sargramostim is produced using a yeast expression system. The modified gene was altered to express a polypeptide with a leucine substitution on the twenty-third position. The purified glycoprotein has 127 amino acids, which are characterized by three primary species with molecular weights of 19.5, 16.8, and 15.5 kDa. The variability in the molecular weight is due to degree of glycosylation. The specific activity of rhGM-CSF is approximately 5.6×10^6 IU/mg.[27]

Pharmacokinetics. Pharmacokinetic profiles have been analyzed in controlled studies of 24 normal male volunteers (Table 5.13). When rhGM-CSF was administered as an intravenous infusion over two hours, the mean elimination half-life was reported as 60 minutes, and the mean clearance rate was observed to be 420 mL/min per square meter. Peak concentrations of GM-CSF were observed in blood samples obtained during or immediately after completion of rhGM-CSF infusion. The mean maximum concentration (Cmax) was 5.0 ng/mL. The mean AUC (0-∞) was 640 ng/mL per minute.[27]

TABLE 5.13. Pharmacokinetics of rhGM-CSF

Pharmacokinetic Parameter	Value
Time to peak levels	1 to 3 h postinjection (SC)
Cmax	5.0 ng/mL (IV)
	1.5 ng/mL (SC)
Clearance rate	420 mL/min per m^2
AUC (0-∞)	640 ng/mL per min
$t_{1/2\beta}$	162 min (SC)

When rhGM-CSF was administered subcutaneously, rhGM-CSF was detected in the serum at 15 minutes, the first sample point. The elimination half-life after a subcutaneous dose was approximately 162 minutes, which is much longer than those reported for intravenous administration. The mean clearance was 529 mL/min per m^2. Peak levels were delayed after SC injection, which occurred at one to three hours postinjection. rhGM-CSF was detectable for up to six hours after SC injection. The Cmax was 1.5 ng/mL after a SC injection. The clearance for subcutaneous injection was similar to intravenous injection, as the mean clearance was 549 mL/min per m^2 and the mean AUC (0-∞) was 549 ng/mL per minute.[27]

Clinical trials in prevention of neutropenia. The ability of rhGM-CSF to accelerate bone marrow recovery has been studied in patients with advanced malignancies and sarcoma. Patients were given varying doses of rhGM-CSF for at least four weeks after they had received their last chemotherapy or radiation treatment. Following initial administration of rhGM-CSF, a transient decrease in absolute neutrophil counts (ANC) persisted in a dose-dependent manner.[28]

The rapid rise of neutrophil is attributed to the rhGM-CSF's ability to mobilize neutrophil progenitors, demargination of neutrophils from blood vessel walls, and prolonged neutrophil survival. The maximal biological effect seemed to occur twice over a 14-day period, as by day five of therapy, the first neutrophil peak increased 1.6- to 4.1-fold. The second peak occurred around day ten, as circulating neutrophils increased 2.2- to 9.7-fold. In contrast to in vitro studies, no consistent elevation of either RBC or platelet counts was seen in these patients. However, a significant increase in both eosinophils and lymphocytes were observed while patients were on rhGM-CSF.

In one study, rhGM-CSF was given at 15 μg/kg per day in patients with small-cell lung cancer (SCLC) treated with a combination of both etoposide and carboplatinum.[29] In this study, the rhGM-CSF therapy was given either for 7, 14, or 21 days. Patients who received rhGM-CSF had lower than expected severe neutropenia (9 percent). This is in contrast to historical controls that reported an incidence of 38 percent of patients developing grade IV neutropenia. This suggests that rhGM-CSF may ameliorate both the duration and severity of neutropenia.

Clinical trials with acute myelogenous leukemia. The safety and efficacy of rhGM-CSF expressed in yeast system was studied in patients with acute myelogenous leukemia (AML). In the phase II study, it was suggested that the best therapeutic effects could be achieved in patients who are at the highest risk for developing severe infections.

Ninety-nine newly diagnosed adult AML patients were evaluated in a multicenter, randomized, double-blind, placebo-controlled study. These patients received a combination of standard doses of daunorubicin (days 1-3) and cytarabine (days 1-7). Patients who were receiving consolidation were given high doses of cytarabine on days one through six. Standard bone marrow evaluation was performed on day ten following induction chemotherapy. In patients whose bone marrow biopsy showed more than 5 percent myeloblasts in the smears, a second cycle of induction chemotherapy was given.

Following chemotherapy, patients were randomly given either rhGM-CSF 250 $\mu g/m^2$ per day or placebo as an intravenous infusion over four hours. rhGM-CSF or placebo was started on the fourth day after the completion of chemotherapy. Drug administration continued until an ANC ($31,500/mm^3$) for three consecutive days, or a maximum of 42 days was achieved.

A patient who received rhGM-CSF had a significantly shortened time when ANC was $< 500/mm^3$ and $< 1,000/mm^3$. In patients receiving rhGM-CSF, ANC $> 500/mm^3$ was achieved by day 16, whereas patients receiving placebo required day 25 to reach the same target. Median times to platelet ($> 20,000/mm^3$) and RBC transfusion independence were not significantly different between treatment groups. During the consolidation phase of treatment, rhGM-CSF did not shorten the median time to recovery of ANC to $500/mm^3$ (13 days) or $1,000/mm^3$ (14.5 days) compared to placebo.

The incidence of severe sickness and deaths associated with infections was significantly reduced in patients who received rhGM-CSF. During induction or consolidation, 27 of 52 patients receiving rhGM-CSF and 35 of 47 patients receiving placebo had at least one grade 3, 4, or 5 infection (p value = 0.02). Twenty-five patients receiving rhGM-CSF and 30 patients receiving placebo experienced severe and fatal infections during induction only. A significant reduction in deaths was attributed to infectious causes in the rhGM-CSF arm (three versus 11, p value = 0.02). In the group receiving placebo, the majority of the deaths were attributed to fungal infections.

The effects of rhGM-CSF on cancer outcomes were also measured. Complete remission (CR) was achieved in 69 percent of the patients receiving rhGM-CSF, whereas only 55 percent CR was seen in patients receiving placebo. Despite improvements in CR outcomes, this difference was not significantly different (p value = 0.21). In addition, no significant difference in relapse rates was seen between the two groups: 12 of 36 patients who received rhGM-CSF and 5 of 26 patients who received placebo relapsed within 180 days of documented CR (p value = 0.26). Overall median survival was 378 days for patients receiving rhGM-CSF, which was not significantly different in patients who received placebo where median survival was 268 days (p value = 0.17).

Clinical trials with autologous bone marrow transplantation. Following a dose-ranging Phase I/II trial in patients undergoing autologous bone marrow transplant (BMT) for lymphoid malignancies, randomized, placebo-controlled, double-blinded studies were conducted to evaluate the safety and efficacy of rhGM-CSF for accelerating hematopoietic reconstitution after autologous BMT.

A total of 128 patients (65 rhGM-CSF, 63 placebo) were enrolled in these studies. The majority of the patients had lymphoid malignancy (87 Non-Hodgkin's Lymphoma [NHL], 17 acute lymphoblastic leukemia [ALL]), 23 patients had Hodgkin's disease, and one patient had acute myeloblastic leukemia (AML). In 72 of the patients with NHL or ALL, the bone marrow harvest was purged prior to storage with one of several monoclonal antibodies. No chemical agent was used for in vitro treatment of the bone marrow. Cytoreductive bone marrow regimens included cyclophosphamide (total dose 120 to 150 mg/kg) and total body irradiation (total dose 1,200 to 1,575 rads). Other regimens used in patients with Hodgkin's disease and NHL without radiotherapy consisted of three or more of the following in combination (expressed as total dose): cytosine arabinoside (400 mg/m^2) and carmustine (300 mg/m^2), cyclophosphamide (140 to 150 mg/kg), hydroxyurea (4.5gm/m^2), and etoposide (375 to 450 mg/m^2).

All three studies tested against placebo were compared with rhGM-CSF. In two of the three studies, improved hematologic indices and clinical end points (e.g., time to neutrophil engraftment, duration of hospitalization and infection experience, or antibacterial usage) were significantly evident. In the third study ($n = 37$), a positive trend toward earlier myeloid engraftment in favor of rhGM-CSF was observed. In the third study, a large number of patients with Hodgkin's disease who had also received extensive radiation and chemotherapy prior to harvest of autologous bone marrow was noted.

A subgroup analysis of the data from all three studies revealed that the median time to engraftment for patients with Hodgkin's disease, regardless of treatment, was six days longer when compared to patients with NHL and ALL, but that the overall beneficial rhGM-CSF treatment effect was the same. In the following combined analysis of the three studies, these two subgroups (NHL and ALL versus Hodgkin's disease) are presented separately.

Myeloid engraftment (ANC 3,500 cells/mm^3) in 54 patients receiving rhGM-CSF was observed six days earlier than in patients receiving placebo. Accelerated myeloid engraftment was associated with significant clinical benefits, as the median duration of hospitalization was six days shorter for the rhGM-CSF group than for the placebo group. Median duration of infectious episodes was three days less in the group treated with rhGM-CSF, which reduced the duration of antibiotic therapy by four days.

Clinical trials with acquired immunodeficiency syndrome. Acquired immunodeficiency syndrome (AIDS) is a viral infection attacking the helper T4 lymphocyte (CD4+), which is the cornerstone of humoral and cellular regulation. Viral infection of CD4+ cells results in altered immune response. Clinical progression will lead to immune system dysfunction, where the cytokine profile will be altered and result in down-regulation of cellular immunity. These changes will place HIV-infected patients at risk for opportunistic infection.[31]

Although the most prominent clinical finding in AIDS patients is a decline in CD4+ cells, the immune responsiveness of myeloid cells is changed due to altered lymphokines when compared to non–HIV-infected patients. rhGM-CSF was given to a patient who had AIDS and leukopenia. A dose-dependent increase in circulating WBC was observed, especially peripheral neutrophils, eosinophils, and monocytes.

A twofold increase in peripheral WBC was seen. In addition, rhGM-CSF was able to reverse neutrophil dysfunction. rhGM-CSF was able to enhance neutrophil activities, such as chemotaxis toward f-Met-Leu-Phe (agent use for in vitro assay for neutrophil chemotactic activity) and increased superoxide production (an indicator of cytotoxic activity). Also noted was an increase in peripheral eosinophils that exceeded the number of mature circulating neutrophils. Although a transient lymphocyte elevation was seen in a few patients, rhGM-CSF did not alter the T4/T8 ratio.

Other studies have confirmed the previous study, in which HIV patients given cytotoxic agents, such as chemotherapy and ganciclovir, were able to benefit from rhGM-CSF. rhGM-CSF is able to ameliorate ganciclovir-induced leukopenia. Subcutaneous injections of rhGM-CSF were given a dose range from 1 to 15 μg/kg per day. Patients receiving doses > 5 μg/kg per day were able to sustain absolute neutrophil counts in the normal range. Peripheral leukocytes were increased 50 to 90 percent above baseline levels, suggesting that rhGM-CSF was able to mitigate myelosuppressive activity of antiviral agents such as ganciclovir. However, some patients experienced an increase of serum p24 when rhGM-CSF was administered, suggesting that rhGM-CSF may activate HIV proliferation.

This was confirmed with an in vitro study in which HIV-infected cells were incubated in the presence of various CSFs. Class I CSF, IL-3, and GM-CSF were able to increase p24, where GM-CSF was able to stimulate the highest level of p24. M-CSF was also able to increase p24, but not at the levels seen with GM-CSF.[32] In contrast, G-CSF had no effect on the p24 levels. This may be due to G-CSF's inability to activate the monotropic HIV cell line (HTLV IIIb), which was used in this study. In addition, GM-CSF and IL-3 have been shown to activate the long terminal repeat (LTR), the promoter of *tat* gene, by increasing transcription of viral proteins.

Conversely, GM-CSF was able to increase the incorporation of zidovudine (AZT) into viral DNA of HIV. Increased AZT incorporation may increase the susceptibility of HIV to antiviral therapy, in which inhibition of HIV replication was attributed to GM-CSF's ability to enhance intracellular phosphorylation of AZT in infected monocytes. rhGM-CSF should be used with caution in patients with HIV. The use of rhGM-CSF in HIV patients should be used in combination with antiretroviral agents.

rhGM-CSF has been used to support WBC counts in AIDS patients receiving chemotherapy. In one study, patients with non-Hodgkin's lymphoma received a regimen containing cyclophosphamide, doxorubicin, vincristine, and prednisone (CHOP). This study randomized patients to receive 10 to 20 μg/kg per day for either days one through ten or four through 13, or no CSFs support at all. No significant difference was seen in patients who were randomized to no CSFs support as compared to patients who received rhGM-CSF from days one through ten. However, in patients who were given rhGM-CSF on days four through 13, a shorter period of neutropenia was seen as compared to no CSF support.[33]

Some studies suggest that GM-CSF can activate HIV replication. In patients receiving rhGM-CSF support, a notable increase of serum p24 was observed, suggesting HIV proliferation during the rhGM-CSF therapy.[34] The p24 levels return to baseline after cessation of rhGM-CSF. Despite an increase in p24, no clinical signs of HIV progression were noted. Therefore, the coadministration of antiviral agents should be encouraged in HIV patients who are receiving rhGM-CSF support.

The standard therapy for HIV-seropositive patients with Kaposi's sarcoma is a combination of interferon-α (IFN-α 1b) and AZT. Unfortunately, patients will develop myelosuppression with long-term therapy. In one study, 19 out of 29 patients developed neutropenia ($< 1,000$ cells/mm^3) requiring rhGM-CSF support. Patients receiving 125 μg/m^2 per day as an SC injection were able to increase ANCs.[35]

rhGM-CSF was also effective in accelerating bone marrow (BM) recovery in HIV patients receiving cytotoxic chemotherapy for either NHL or Kaposi's sarcoma. Bone marrow suppressive effects were ameliorated with the use of rhG-CSF and were similar to that of rhGM-CSF. Unlike some patients who received rhGM-CSF, there was no elevation of serum p24 in these patients.

Adverse reactions. An acute toxicity study revealed an absence of treatment-related toxicity following a single IV bolus injection at a dose of 300 μg/kg. Two subacute studies were performed using IV injection (maximum dose 200 μg/kg per day × 14 days) and subcutaneous injection (maximum dose 200 μg/kg per day × 28 days). No major visceral organ toxicity was documented. Notable histopathology findings included increased cellularity in hematologic organs, and in heart and lung tissues. A dose-dependent increase in leukocyte count, which consisted primarily of segmented neutrophils, occurred during the dosing period; increases in monocytes, basophils, eosinophils, and lymphocytes were also noted. Leukocyte counts decreased to pretreatment values over a recovery period of one to two weeks.

Erythropoietin

Erythropoietin (EPO) is a glycoprotein produced primarily by kidney cells in response to low blood oxygen tension. This glycoprotein is a hematopoietic growth factor that governs the terminal maturation and differentiation of erythroid progenitors. Basal levels of EPO in normal subjects ranges from 0.01 to 0.03 U/mL; however, levels can increase 100 to 1,000-fold of baseline during episodes of hypoxia anemia.

In patients with chronic renal failure (CRF), kidney cells are unable to produce adequate amounts of EPO, which will lead to anemia. Patients with chronic renal failure will have progressive decline in kidney function as measured by glomerular filtration decline with accompanying anemia.

Epoetin alfa (Epogen®/Procrit®)

Product information. Epoetin alfa (recombinant EPO) has been approved to treat anemia associated with chronic renal failure (CRF) for patients by at least maintaining or elevating hematocrit or hemoglobin levels.[36] Recombinant human EPO is produced by the insertion of the EPO gene into the chinese hamster ovary (CHO) mammalian expression system. The purified product is a glycoprotein with 165 amino acids, with a molecular weight of 30 kDa. Since full glycosylation is required for full EPO biological activity, only a mammalian expression system with the necessary cellular machinery for posttranslational modification is able to produce biologically active EPO.[36]

When CRF patients with anemia are given EPO, erythropoiesis is stimulated and circulating hemoglobulin and hematocrit levels improve with continued use. The first evidence of clinical response is a rise in circulating reticulocytes, which are precursors of mature erythrocyte or red blood cells (RBC). The timing of the response is usually within ten days from the initiation of therapy. Maturation of reticulocytes to RBC is evident by increases in hemoglobin and hematocrit, which are apparent within two to six weeks. Once the hematocrit reaches the target range (30 to 36 percent), that level can be sustained by erythropoietin therapy in the absence of iron deficiency and concurrent illnesses.

Pharmacokinetics. Intravenously administered rhEPO is eliminated at a rate consistent with first-order kinetics with a circulating half-life ranging from approximately four to 13 hours in patients with CRF. Within the therapeutic dose range, detectable levels of plasma erythropoietin are maintained for at least 24 hours.[36] When rhEPO is administered subcutaneously in patients with CRF, peak serum levels are achieved within five to 24 hours after administration. There is a difference in the elimination half-life between patients not on dialysis as compared to those who are maintained on dialysis. When compared to normal volunteers, the elimination half-life after an IV dose of rhEPO is approximately 20 percent shorter than the half-life in CRF patients.[37]

Clinical trials with chronic renal failure. Response to rhEPO was consistent across all studies. In the presence of adequate iron stores, the time to reach the target hematocrit (Hct) is a function of the baseline hematocrit and the rate of hematocrit rise. The rate of increase in Hct is dependent upon the dose of rhEPO administered.

Over this dose range of 50 to 150 U/kg three times per week, approximately 95 percent of all patients responded clinically as evident by an increase in Hct; virtually all patients were transfusion independent after two months of therapy. In addition, patients receiving rhEPO showed a statistically significant increase in exercise capacity (VO_2 max), energy, and strength.

From clinical studies involving CRF patients requiring chronic dialysis, the median maintenance dose to maintain a Hct between 30 and 36 percent was 75 U/kg three times per week. A multicenter unit dose study was also conducted in 119 patients receiving peritoneal dialysis who self-administered rhEPO subcutaneously and responded in a manner similar to patients receiving IV administration.

In a study involving 181 patients with CRF not requiring dialysis, they were given rhEPO in a manner similar to that observed in patients on dialysis. Similar to other CRF patients, rhEPO showed a dose-dependent increase of Hct. Moreover, rhEPO doses of 75 to 150 U/kg per week have been shown to maintain hematocrits of 36 to 38 percent for up to six months.

Clinical trials with zidovudine-treated HIV-infected patients. Responsiveness to EPO in HIV-infected patients is dependent upon the endogenous serum erythropoietin level prior to treatment. Patients with endogenous serum EPO levels < 500 MU/mL, and who are receiving a dose of zidovudine < 4,200 mg/week, may respond to EPO therapy. In contrast, patients with endogenous serum EPO levels > 500 MU/mL do not appear to respond to rhEPO therapy. In a series of four clinical trials, 60 to 80 percent of HIV-infected patients treated with zidovudine (AZT) had endogenous serum erythropoietin levels < 500 MU/mL. These patients showed reduced transfusion requirements and increased Hct.[38]

Clinical trials with cancer patients on chemotherapy. Anemia in cancer patients can be related to the disease and the administration of cytotoxic chemotherapy. Patients who were treated with chemotherapy had varying levels of endogenous EPO. It was found that 83 out of 110 (75 percent) patients had serum EPO levels < 132 MU/mL and only 4 out of 110 (4 percent) had endogenous serum EPO levels > 500 MU/mL. In general, patients with lower baseline serum EPO levels were more responsive to rhEPO when compared to patients with higher baseline endogenous levels of erythroid growth factor.

In one double-blinded placebo controlled trial in which 131 anemic cancer patients were enrolled, 72 patients were treated with concomitant noncisplatin-containing chemotherapy regimens and 59 patients were treated with concomitant cisplatin-containing chemotherapy regimens. Patients were randomly assigned to receive either rhEPO 150 U/kg or placebo subcutaneously three times per week for 12 weeks.[36]

Patients receiving rhEPO had a significantly greater response as compared to the placebo-controlled group (p value < 0.008). After the first month of therapy, the number of units of blood (0.71 versus 1.84 units) transfused per patient was significantly reduced (p value < 0.02) compared to control group. The reduction of transfusion was observed with continual therapy in months 2 and 3.

Clinical trials with surgery patients. rhEPO has been studied in a placebo-controlled, double-blind trial that involved 316 patients who were scheduled for major elective orthopedic hip or knee surgery. Patients requiring more than two units of blood were enrolled in this study. Patients were stratified into one of three groups based on their pretreatment hemoglobin [<10 ($n = 2$), >10 to <13 ($n = 96$), and >13 to <15 g/dL ($n = 218$)] and then randomly assigned to receive 300 U/kg EPO, 100 U/kg EPO, or placebo by SC injection for ten days before surgery, on the day of surgery, and for four days after surgery.[36]

Patients with a baseline Hgb (Hemoglobin) between 10 to 13 g/dL receiving rhEPO 300 U/kg reduced the need for allogeneic transfusion. There was no significant difference in the number of patients transfused between the various groups whose baseline Hgb was 13 to 15 g/dL.

rhEPO was also studied in an open-label, parallel-group trial enrolling 145 subjects with a pretreatment Hgb 10 to 13 g/dL who were scheduled for major orthopedic hip or knee surgery and were not participating in an autologous program. Subjects were randomly assigned to receive one of two SC dosing regimens of EPO (600 U/kg once weekly for three weeks prior to surgery and on the day of surgery, or 300 U/kg once daily for ten days prior to surgery, on the day of surgery, and for four days after surgery).

Adverse reactions. EPO therapy is associated with some serious adverse effects that require careful patient monitoring. Reports of hypertension in anemia patients with chronic renal failure have been documented. The risk for hypertension appears to be related to a wide variety of factors including concurrent EPO therapy, an increase in hematocrit, increased blood viscosity, and a decrease in hypoxic vasodilation.[36] Patients with a preexisting history of hypertension may require dose escalation in antihypertensive therapy.

Seizures have also occurred during EPO therapy that may be related to a sudden increase in blood pressure associated with an increase in hematocrit. Patients should be monitored for hematocrit levels and headaches. A rise in hematocrit greater than 4 percent in any two-week period requires an immediate reduction in dose of EPO.[36]

Other adverse effects associated with EPO therapy include thrombophlebitis as a result of clotting problems arising from an increased blood viscosity, a rise in platelet counts, and a decrease in bleeding time.[36] Reports of fever, myalgia, weakness, nausea, vomiting, diarrhea, and hyperkalemia have been documented.

Dosage and administration. Prior to initiating EPO therapy, baseline blood levels of EPO should be obtained to confirm that anemia is associated with low EPO levels. The dose of EPO ranges from 50 to 300 U/kg given three times a week, which will influence the rate of erythropoiesis. At doses greater than 300 U/kg, no dose-dependent biological responses have been shown.[37] Other factors affecting the rate and extent of response include availability of iron, which is required for biosynthesis of hemoglobulin. Patients undergoing EPO therapy may develop absolute or functional iron deficiencies if iron supplementation is not coadministered. Iron supplementation is usually administered in the form of ferrous sulfate 325 mg three times per day, then is reduced as target hemoglobin is reached. The adult target hemoglobin in males ranges from 13.5 to 17.5 g/dL and 12 to 16 g/dL in females. The normal adult hematocrit in males ranges from 41 to 53 percent and 36 to 46 percent in females.[39] Functional iron deficiency is characterized with low transferrin saturation associated with an inability to adequately mobilize iron with increased erythropoiesis.[37] Thus, transferrin saturation and serum ferritin levels should be monitored at baseline and during EPO therapy. Thrombotic events have been associated with patients with high hematocrit during EPO therapy.

PLATELET-DERIVED GROWTH FACTOR BB

Diabetes mellitus affects over 16 million Americans.[40] Two common complications associated with diabetes are neuropathy and peripheral vascular disease (PVD). These two complications increase the risk of developing cutaneous ulcers.[41] Diabetic foot ulcers often start as a result of minor trauma characterized by a loss of epithelium. The injury can extend beyond borders of the initial trauma and can involve the dermal layer.[42] Besides predisposing patients to developing foot ulcers, peripheral neuropathy and PVD also impede wound healing and closure as a consequence of poor vascularization.[42,43,44] The open wound along with ischemia from PVD allows for bacterial seeding and proliferation, which can lead to systemic infection.[41]

A number of factors regulate the wound-healing process. One of these factors is platelet-derived growth factor (PDGF). The biological activity of PDGF has been indicated to promote the synthesis and migration of proteins.[45] PDGF and extracellular matrix components such as lamina can stimulate fibroblasts, smooth muscle cells, and capillary endothelial cells. PDGF can also promote cell chemotaxis and activation of inflammatory cells.[46]

PDGF is a dimer consisting of two polypeptides, referred to as A and B subunits. Three forms of PDGF have been described and are classified as PDGF-AA, PDGF-AB, and PDGF-BB.[43] Although all of these isoforms are biologically active, fibroblast cells seem to be the most responsive to PDGF-BB.[43]

Becaplermin (Regranex®)

Product Information

Becaplermin is a recombinant human platelet-derived growth factor (rhPDGF-BB) that is indicated for the treatment of diabetic foot ulcers in the lower extremities extending into the subcutaneous tissues or beyond.[47] This product is produced with recombinant DNA technology by inserting the gene encoding for the B chain of PDGF into a yeast expression system, *Saccharomyces cerevisiae*. The expressed product is a homodimer composed of two identical polypeptides with an approximate molecular weight of 25 kDa. The chains are held together by intrachain disulfide bonds. Becaplermin is suspended in a buffered, aqueous-based carboxymethylcellulose (NaCMC) gel. It has activity similar to that of endogenous PDGF-BB, including accelerating the wound-healing cascade and promoting the formation of granulation tissue.[47]

Becaplermin is a clear, colorless gel containing 100 μg of becaplermin per gram of gel. The product should be refrigerated at 2° to 8°C (36° to 46°F) but not frozen or used after the expiration date.[47]

Pharmacokinetics

Systemic absorption of becaplermin gel was examined in multiple clinical trials. Plasma PDGF-BB levels remained at or near baseline for most of the study patients, even after 14 days of therapy.[47] Systemic bioavailability was determined to be approximately 3 percent in full-thickness wounds receiving single or multiple daily applications.[47]

Clinical Trials

Becaplermin was evaluated in a multicenter, double-blinded, placebo-controlled phase III trial, involving 382 patients with confirmed diabetic foot ulcers. Entry criteria required that ulcers were at least eight weeks in duration. These patients were randomized to receive one of the following: becaplermin gel 30 μg/g, becaplermin gel 100 μg/g, or placebo gel. The regimen was combined with good wound care and continued until complete wound closure or a maximum of 20 weeks.

The results showed that becaplermin gel 100 μg/g increased the incidence of complete wound closure by 43 percent compared to placebo (50 percent versus 35 percent).[47] Also, becaplermin 100 μg/g gel reduced the time to achieve complete wound healing by 32 percent (86 versus 127 days).[47] In groups treated with becaplermin 30 μg/g, 36 percent of patients achieved complete wound healing, compared to 35 percent in the placebo group.[44] The safety profile of becaplermin gel was found to be similar to that of placebo gel.

Another randomized, double-blinded, placebo-controlled trial evaluated the efficacy of becaplermin in 118 patients with chronic, nonhealing, full-thickness lower extremity ulcers. Patients were randomized to receive becaplermin gel 2.2 μg/cm^2 every 24 hours or placebo for 20 weeks or until complete wound closure.[44] Results showed that 48 percent of patients in the becaplermin group achieved complete wound healing during the study period, compared to only 25 percent in the placebo group. Also the reduction in wound area was 98.8 percent in the becaplermin group compared to 82.1 percent in the placebo group.[44]

Adverse Reactions

Results of six clinical trials comparing becaplermin gel, placebo, and good ulcer care alone showed a 2 percent incidence of erythematous rash associated with becaplermin use.[47] Many other adverse events, including osteomyelitis, infection, and cellulitis, were reported in similar incidences as placebo.[47]

Dosage and Administration

Becaplermin is available in 2, 7.5, and 15 g tubes. The amount of gel applied will depend on the size of the ulcer area.[47] Once measured, the gel should be spread evenly (approximately 1/16 inch) over the entire area of the wound. The site of application should be covered with a saline-moistened dressing for 12 hours. Once cleaned, the wound should be kept covered with just a saline dressing for the remainder of the day. Becaplermin should be applied once daily until the wound is completely healed.[47]

NOTES

1. Louie SG, Jung B. Clinical effects of biological response modifiers. *Am J Hosp Pharm* 1993;50:S10-S18.

2. Product Information. Aldesleukin. Emeryville, CA: Chiron Corp, 1999.

3. Konrad MS, Hemstreet G, Hersh EM, Mansell PWA, Mertelsman R, Lolitz JE, Bradley EC. Pharmacokinetics of recombinant interleukin-2 in humans. *Cancer Res* 1900;50:2009-2017.

4. Rosenberg SA, Lotze MT, Muul LM, Chang AE, Avis FP, Leitman S, Linehan WM, Robertson CN, Lee RE, Rubin JT., et al. A progress report on the treatment of 157 patients with advanced cancer using lymphokine-activated killer cells and interleukin-2 or high-dose interleukin-2 alone. *N Engl J Med* 1987; 316:889-897.

5. Rosenberg SA, Lotze MT, Muul LM, Leitman S, Chang AE, Ettinghausen SE, Matory YL, Skibber JM, Shiloni E, Vetto JT, et al. Observations on the systemic administration of autologous lymphokine-activated killer cells and recombinant interleukin-2 to patients with metastatic cancer. *N Engl J Med* 1985;313:1485-1492.

6. Gordon MS, McCaskill-Stevens WJ, Battiato LA, et al. A phase I trial of recombinant human interleukin-11 (neumega rhIL-11 growth factor) in women with breast cancer receiving chemotherapy. *Blood* 1996;87:3615-3624.

7. Tepler I, Elias L, Smith II JW, et al. A randomized placebo-controlled trial of recombinant human interleukin-11 in cancer patients with severe thrombocytopenia due to chemotherapy. *Blood* 1996;87:3607-3614.

8. Wallace EL, Churchill WH, Surgenor DM, et al. Collection and transfusion of blood and blood components in the United States, 1992. *Transfusion* 1995; 35:802.

9. Product Information: Neumega, Oprelvekin. Genetics Institute, Cambridge, MA, 1998.

10. Kobayashi S, Teramura M, Oshimi K, Mizoguchi H. Interleukin-11. *Leuk Lymph* 1994;15:45-49.

11. Teramura M, Kobayashi S, Hoshino S, et al. Interleukin-11 enhances human megakaryocytopoiesis in vitro. *Blood* 1992;79:327-331.

12. Orazi A, Cooper RJ, Tong J, et al. Effects of recombinant human interleukin-11 on megakaryocytopoiesis in human bone marrow. *Exp Hematol* 1996;24:1289-1297.

13. Musashi M, Yang YC, Paul S, et al. Direct and synergistic effects of interleukin-11 on murine hemopoiesis in culture. *Proc Natl Acad Sci USA* 1991; 88:765-769.

14. Peterson RL, Wang L, Albert L. Molecular effects of recombinant human interleukin-11 in the HLA-B27 rat model of inflammatory bowel disease. *Lab Invest* 1998;78:1503-1512.

15. Aoyama K, Uchida T, Takanuki F, et al. Pharmacokinetics of recombinant human interleukin-11 (rhIL-11) in healthy male subjects. *Brit J Clin Pharm* 1997; 43:571-578.

16. Shen WC, Louie SG. *Immunology for pharmacists and pharmaceutical scientists*, Harwood Press, 1998.

17. AHFS Drug information 96. Bethesda, MD: American Society of Health-System Pharmacists, Inc., 1996;775-804.

18. Fauci AS, Rosenberg SA, Sherwin SA, et al. Immunomodulators in clinical medicine. *Ann Internal Med* 1987;106:421-433.

19. Product Information: Roferon A. Nutley, NJ: Hoffman La-Roche, 1999.

20. Product Information: Intron A. Kenilworth, NJ: Schering Corp, 1999.

21. Product Information: Interferon alfacon-1. Thousand Oaks, CA: Amgen, Inc., 1999.

22. Gill PS, Masood R, Cai J, Louie SG, Harrington W, Lin G, Law R, Levine AM. Novel antiviral therapy for HTLV-I associated acute T-cell leukemia. *Blood* 1992;80:74.

23. Product Information: Avenox. Cambridge, MA, 1999.

24. Product Information: Betaseron. Emeryville, CA, 1999.

25. Product Information: Actimmune. Brisbane, CA, 1999.

26. Product Information: Filgrastim. Thousand Oaks, CA: Amgen, Inc., 1999.

27. Product Information: Sargramostim. Seattle, WA: Immunex Corp, 1999.

28. Neumunaitis J, Rabinowe SN, Singer JW, Bierman PJ, Vose JM, Freedman AS, Onetto N, Gillis S, Oette D, Gold M. Recombinant granulocyte-macrophage colony-stimulating factor after autologous bone marrow transplantation for lymphoid cancer. *New Eng J Med* 1991;324(25):1773-1778.

29. Luikart SD, Herndon JE, Hollis DR, MacDonald M, Maurer LH, Crawford J, Clamon GH, Wright J, Perry MC, Ozer H, Green MR. Phase I trial of etoposide, carboplatin, and GM-CSF in extensive small-cell lung cancer: A cancer and leukemia group B study (CALGB 8832). *Am J Clin Onc* 1997;20(1):24-30.

30. Carlo-Stella C, Regazzi E, Andrizzi C, Savoldo B, Garau D, Montefusco E, Vignetti M, Mandelli F, Rizzoli V, Meloni G. Use of granulocyte-macrophage colony-stimulating factor (GM-CSF) in combination with hydroxyurea as post-transplant therapy in chronic myelogenous leukemia patients autografted with unmanipulated hematopoietic cells. *Haematologica* 1997;82(3):291-296.

31. Groopman JE, Mitsuyasu RT, DeLeo MJ, Oette DH, Golde DW. Effect of recombinant human granulocyte-macrophage colony-stimulating factor on myelopoiesis in the acquired immunodeficiency syndrome. *New Eng J Med* 1987;317 (10):593-598.

32. Koyanagi Y, O'Brien WA, Zhao JQ, Golde DW, Gasson JC, Chen IS. Cytokines alter production of HIV-1 from primary mononuclear phagocytes. *Science* 1988;241(4873):1673-1675.

33. Perno CF, Yarchoan R, Cooney DA, Hartman NR, Webb DS, Hao Z, Mitsuya H, Johns DG, Broder S. Replication of human immunodeficiency virus in monocytes. Granulocyte/macrophage colony-stimulating factor (GM-CSF) potentiates viral production yet enhances the antiviral effect mediated by 3'-azido-2'3'-dideoxythymidine (AZT) and other dideoxynucleoside congeners of thymidine. *J Eperimental Med* 1989;169(3):933-951.

34. Straus DJ. Prognostic factors in the treatment of human immunodeficiency virus-associated non-Hodgkin's lymphoma. *Recent Results in Cancer Research* 2002;159:143-148.

35. Kaplan LD, Kahn JO, Crowe S, Northfelt D, Neville P, Grossberg H, Abrams DI, Tracey J, Mills J, Voldberding PA. Clinical and virologic effects of recombinant human granulocyte-macrophage colony-stimulating factor in patients receiving chemotherapy for human immunodeficiency virus-associated non-Hodgkin's lymphoma: Results of a randomized trial. *J Clin Onc* 1991;9(6):929-940.

36. Clinical Pharmacology. Product Information: Epoetin alfa. Thousand Oaks, CA, 1999.

37. Product Information: Epoetin alfa. Thousand Oaks, CA: Amgen Inc., 1999.

38. Miles SA, Mitsuyasu RT, Moreno J, Baldwin G, Alton NK, Souza L, Glaspy JA. Combined therapy with recombinant granulocyte colony-stimulating factor and erythropoietin decreases hematologic toxicity from zidovudine. *Blood* 1991; 77(10):2109-2117.

39. Dipiro JT, Talbert RL, Yee GC, et al. Thromboembolic disorders. In Erdman SM, Rodvold KA, Friedenberg WR (Eds.), *Pharmacotherapy: A pathophysiologic approach,* Third edition. Stamford, CT: Appleton & Lange, 1997.

40. National Diabetes Fact Sheet. Atlanta, GA: U.S. Department of Health and Human Services, Public Health Services, 1997.

41. Weiman TJ. Clinical efficacy of becaplermin (rhPDGF-BB) gel. *Am J Surg* 1998;176:74S-79S.

42. Reiber GE, Lipsky BA, Gibbons GW. The burden of diabetic foot ulcers. *Am J Surg* 1998;176:5S-10S.

43. Smiell JM. Clinical safety of becaplermin (rhPDGF-BB) gel. *Am J Surg* 1998;(Supp 2A):68S-73S.

44. Weiman TJ, Smiell JM, Su Y. Efficacy and safety of a topical gel formulation of recombinant human platelet-derived growth factor-BB (Becaplermin) in patients with chronic neuropathic diabetic foot ulcers: A phase III randomized placebo-controlled double-blind study. *Diabetes Care* 1998;21:822-827.

45. LeGrand E. Preclinical promise of becaplermin (rhPDGF-BB) in wound healing. *Am J Surg* 1998;176(Supp 2A):48S-54S.

46. Ross R. Peptide regulatory factors: Platelet-derived growth factor. *Lancet* 1989;1:1179-1182.

47. Product Information: Regranex, Becaplermin. Ortho-McNeil Pharmaceuticals, Raritan, NJ, 1998.

Chapter 6

Anticytokines

Stan G. Louie
Jay P. Rho
Amir Aminimanizani
Parul Patel

INTRODUCTION

Cytokines, literally translated as cell growth factors, are actually proteins or glycoproteins that can stimulate or inhibit the activation of various biological responses. Physiologically, a stimulatory signal must be balanced with the presence of an inhibitory or down-regulatory signal. An inability to down-regulate a signal may present a problem, such as increased tissue injury. Examples of signal dysregulation include septic shock and autoimmune diseases. Both of these scenarios represent an inability to down-regulate the immune system. This is evident by an overproduction of inflammatory mediators such as interleukin-1 (IL-1) and tumor necrosis factor (TNF). These cytokines, in turn, stimulate the production of other cytokines and prostaglandin synthesis, thus activating a cascade of biological activity.

The body is able to sustain tissue injury for a short period of time. When prolonged periods of tissue injury persist, serious clinical manifestations can occur. This may be due to the persistence of antigens or an inability to down-regulate the activated immune system. It has been shown that the addition of cytokine modulators may be able to ameliorate tissue damage due to an exaggerated immune response.[1,2]

Anticytokines are immune modulating factors produced by the body. These factors exist in two major classifications, antagonist ligands and soluble receptors. Both of these factors inhibit ligand-receptor binding, thus blocking the intracellular signals that propagate the activated state. In essence, anticytokines act as modulators that switch off an immune response.

INTERLEUKIN-1 RECEPTOR ANTAGONIST

IL-1 inhibitory activity was first observed in the supernatants of monocytes cultured on adherent immunoglobulins (IgG). Later, a factor isolated from the urine of febrile patients was found to have similar biological activity. This protein was later called interleukin-1 receptor antagonist (IL-1ra). IL-1ra is a naturally occurring glycoprotein that competitively inhibits the binding of both interleukin-1α and β (IL-1α and IL-1β) onto the IL-1 receptor (IL-1r).[3] Unlike other IL-1 receptor ligands, IL-1ra does not initiate any intracellular signals leading to protein transcription. Instead, the lack of stimulatory properties suggests that IL-1ra is a competitive inhibitor of IL-1α and β (Figure 6.1).

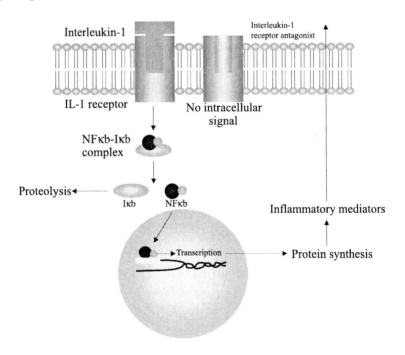

FIGURE 6.1. Mechanism of IL-1ra transcription blockade

Keratinocytes and other epithelial cells produce a second form of IL-1ra created from an alternative splicing reaction of ribonucleic acid. This protein is synthesized without a leader sequence, but possesses seven additional amino acid residues at the amino terminus in comparison with the extracellular monocyte form of IL-1ra.[1,2,3] The keratinocyte variant of IL-1ra remains cell associated and has been termed intracellular IL-1ra, or icIL-1ra.

Pharmacology

IL-1ra exerts its biological activity by competitively binding onto Type I IL-1r. The binding affinity of IL-1ra onto the Type 1 IL-1r is equal to that of IL-1α and IL-1β, but it has a lower affinity for the Type II IL-1r than IL-1β.[3] The similarity in binding affinity is attributed to the fact that IL-1ra is a member of the IL-1 family with 26 percent amino acid sequence homology to IL-1β and 19 percent to IL-1α. Extracellular IL-1ra from monocytes exists as a 17 kDa non-glycosylated molecule and as variably glycosylated forms, 22 to 25 kDa in weight. When given at 30 molar excess above IL-1 concentration, complete blockade is achieved.

IL-1ra is released during inflammation in response to various natural disorders.[4] It is a natural regulatory mechanism designed to prevent overstimulation resulting in deleterious effects from IL-1.[5,6] In animal models, pretreatment with IL-1ra is able to prevent death caused by excessive lipopolysaccharide (LPS)-induced septic shock syndrome.[7] LPS was able to induce expression of both IL-1 and TNF.[8] Other potential uses of IL-1ra include autoimmune diseases that develop in response to high cytokine elaboration, such as inflammatory bowl disease.[9] In this arena, the absence of IL-1ra is thought to play a role in human inflammatory bowel disease.[10]

Pharmacokinetics

The pharmacokinetics of IL-1ra was evaluated in 25 healthy male volunteers from 18 to 30 years of age. IL-1ra was administered as a three-hour continuous infusion in a dose ranging from 1 to 10 mg/kg. Plasma IL-1ra levels were 3.1 μg/ml and 29 μg/ml for the 1 mg/kg and 10 mg/kg doses, respectively. Following dosage administration,

IL-1ra levels exhibiting a biphase decline with an initial half-life of 21 minutes, and a terminal half-life of 108 minutes.[11]

Clinical Trials

Deaths attributed to septic shock are a leading cause of mortality in the United States. Septic shock syndrome is initiated by the presence of bacterial antigen, usually from a gram-negative species, in the circulation, which causes bacteremia. Although it may occur with gram-positive organisms, such as *Staphylococcus aureus* (as in toxic shock syndrome), the syndrome is normally activated by the presence of lipopolysaccharides (LPS) or endotoxins that are present on the surface of gram-negative organisms.[12]

LPS has been shown to be a potent stimulator of immune activation. In fact, septic syndrome may be described as an exaggerated immune response to the antigen resulting in an overproduction of inflammatory mediators such as TNF and IL-1.[13] During a septic episode, massive quantities of IL-1 and TNF are produced. In fact, serum concentrations of TNF can transiently exceed 10^{-7} M.[13]

IL-1 is a primary growth factor that activates the entire immune system. It has myriad biological activities, which include mobilization of white blood cells (WBCs), induction of adrenocorticotropic hormone (ACTH), and induction of cytokine expression. Physiologically, the administration of IL-1 can cause flulike symptoms, such as fever, chills, rigors, myalgias, and arthralgias. The ability to induce these physiological responses has coined IL-1 as an endogenous pyrogen.[1,2]

The treatment of septic shock induced by gram-negative bacteria involves the elimination of immune activation. Thus, LPS-directed antibodies may be able to prevent the onset of septic shock syndrome. Two monoclonal antibodies have been tested in humans to prevent septic shock. Because these agents are not FDA approved, the current treatment is supportive care.

Supportive care begins with hemodynamic support, such as fluid challenge. If fluid challenge is unable to reverse TNF-induced hypotension, the use of β-adrenergic agonists, such as dopamine and dobutamine, may be necessary. Adequate maintenance of blood pressure may retain sufficient organ perfusion. Monitoring for normalization of laboratory values (i.e., liver function tests, serum creatinine, cardiac ejection fraction) is important.[13]

Although aggressive supportive care may be important in the acute phase of the syndrome, the elimination of LPS is sentinel in determining clinical outcome. This may be accomplished by using appropriate antibiotics active against the pathogen. Steroids can also be used to prevent or ameliorate septic shock caused by LPS. Other drugs, such as naloxone, have been explored for potential use but with no clinically significant outcomes. Thus, current treatment relies on effective antibiotic coverage and aggressive supportive care.

Future therapeutic options will be to immunomodulate primary inflammatory mediators such as TNF and IL-1. This can be accomplished by generating monoclonal antibodies directed against these cytokines. In addition, the isolation of competitive antagonists (i.e., IL-1ra) has been shown in clinical trials to be safe and effective in ameliorating septic shock syndrome. In the future, eliciting point mutations in RNA coding for the native protein will produce custom competitive antagonists.

A large amount of evidence indicates that both IL-1 and TNF-α are important mediators in animal models of overwhelming sepsis and shock.[1,2,3] The relative importance of each cytokine has been somewhat difficult to discern because both IL-1 and TNF-α are capable of inducing the production of themselves or the other cytokine. The endogenous production of IL-1ra in primates with septic shock, although considerable, is inadequate to counteract the stimulating effects of IL-1.

Inflammation in mice or rats induced by the in vivo injection of bacterial LPS requires constant or repeated administration of IL-1ra to yield significant inhibition. IL-1ra is effective in markedly decreasing mortality in mice, rats, or rabbits with septic shock induced by large amounts of LPS.[1,2,3,6] In each instance, however, IL-1ra had to be given concurrently or shortly after LPS administration. More recent studies indicate that the effects of IL-1ra vary considerably in animals with sepsis, depending on many factors, such as the amount of LPS or live organism used, and the timing and amount of IL-1ra administered. IL-1ra markedly attenuates the hemodynamic markers of shock after injection with a lethal dose of *E. coli* in baboons.[14]

The results of recent studies describe some further possible beneficial effects of IL-1ra in infections. In addition to effects in gram-negative sepsis, IL-1ra attenuates the hemodynamic abnormalities and decreases the endogenous production of IL-1 and TNFα in a rabbit model of gram-negative sepsis secondary to *Staphylococcus epidermidis*.

Adverse Reactions

Clinical, hematological, biochemical, endocrinological, and immunomodulatory effects were monitored over 72 hours and compared to those of four subjects receiving a three-hour infusion of saline. No clinically significant differences were found between the drug and saline groups in symptoms, physical examinations, complete blood counts, mononuclear cell phenotypes, blood chemistry profiles, serum iron, and serum cortisol levels. Peripheral blood mononuclear cells (PBMCs) obtained after completion of the IL-1ra infusion synthesized significantly less IL-6 ex vivo than PBMCs from saline-injected controls. These data suggest that transient blockade of IL-1ra is safe and does not significantly affect homeostasis.

Dosage and Administration

IL-1ra is still under investigation. Dosage or administration of this drug is under the guidelines set forth by the FDA.

TUMOR NECROSIS FACTOR SOLUBLE RECEPTOR

Soluble TNF was first discovered when bacterial extracts were injected into tumor-bearing mice resulting in a reduction of tumor size. Investigators studying factors affecting appetite discovered a soluble factor capable of decreasing appetite which they termed *cachectin*. It was later found that cachectin and TNF were the same molecule.[13]

Similar to IL-1, TNF acts as an endogenous pyrogen that is able to induce fevers via stimulation of the hypothalamic region in the brain. Fevers may be prolonged by TNF and IL-1's ability to increase synthesis of prostaglandins. Other pluritropic activities of TNF include stimulating the production of other inflammatory mediators, such as IL-2 and IL-6, and causing flulike symptoms. In addition, elevated levels of TNF can cause vascular dilation, manifesting as hypotension, and a decrease in appetite resulting in weight loss.

TNF-mediated injuries may result in an increase in capillary leakage, leading to decreased intravascular volume. The body will compensate for the drop in blood pressure by inducing tachycardia. However, a second deleterious effect of TNF is its ability to depress myocardial contractility, which can decrease the effectiveness of reflex tachycardia compensating for decreased intravascular volume. Furthermore, TNF is able to reduce blood pressure and tissue profusion by relaxing vascular smooth muscle tone. This reduction of muscle tone can be mediated via direct or indirect TNF stimulation of endothelial cells to produce vasodilators, such as prostacycline, and activate nitric oxide synthetase to increase production of nitric oxide. TNF-mediated coagulation and activation of neutrophils leading to vascular plugging can further decrease organ perfusion.

The major cellular source of TNF in septic shock is from the LPS-activated mononuclear phagocyte (macrophage), although antigen stimulated T-cells, activated NK cells, and activated mast cells can also enhance production of this cytokine. Interferon gamma (IFN-γ), produced by T-cells, augments TNF synthesis in LPS-stimulated monocytes. Thus, TNF is a mediator of both natural and acquired immunity.

The biological activity of TNF is best understood at low concentrations. TNF can cause vascular endothelial cells to become adhesive for leukocytes, initially for neutrophils, and subsequently for monocytes and lymphocytes. These actions contribute to the accumulation of leukocytes at local sites of inflammation. Furthermore, TNF is able to stimulate macrophages to produce cytokines, including IL-1, interleukin-6 (IL-6), TNF itself, and interleukin-8 (IL-8). Other TNF effects include stimulation of vascular endothelial cells and fibroblasts to produce colony-stimulating factors (or myeloid growth factors, CSFs).

Similar to TNF, IL-1 is a primary inflammatory mediator, which is produced by stimulated monocytes. Also similar to TNF, LPS activation of monocytes can increase synthesis and secretion of IL-1. IL-1 is different from TNF in two regards. First, IL-1 is able to stimulate CD4+ cells and cellular production of IL-1. Second, IL-1 has been shown to increase transcription of the IL-2 gene. IL-1 can also stimulate monocytes and endothelial cells to produce IL-1 and IL-6. In general, slight differences between IL-1 and TNF exist; however, their biological activities are very similar.

TNF-α has two types of soluble receptors, which are designated by their molecular weight of 55 kDa and 75 kDa. These two soluble receptors are more commonly referred to as p55 and p75 or receptors I and II. Both soluble receptors can bind onto TNF, thus reduce the levels of TNF available for cellular binding and immune activation. Numerous anticytokines are now being evaluated for clinical use. These are reviewed in Table 6.1.

Rheumatoid Arthritis

Rheumatoid arthritis (RA) affects approximately 1 percent of the U.S. population (2.5 million). A chronic autoimmune disorder, RA usually presents with destruction of peripheral bone, joints, and cartilage. Radiographic findings usually reveal progressive erosion of bone and cartilage with regional bony decalcification. Other clinical features include synovial hypertrophy, with fluid and inflammatory cell infiltration. Systemic features of this immune disorder can include a marked acute phase response and the production of auto-antibodies.[15]

The primary site of damage occurs at the junction of the synovium lining, the affected joint capsule with bone and cartilage. The af-

TABLE 6.1. Anticytokine Agents

Target Cytokine	Anticytokine
TNF-α	Anti-TNF antibody
	Soluble p55 receptor
	p55-IgG$_1$ fusion protein
	Soluble p75 receptor
	p75-IgG$_1$ Fc fusion protein
	TNF converting enzyme inhibitor
Interleukin-1	Interleukin-1 receptor antagonist
	Interleukin-1 type I soluble receptor
	Interleukin-1 type II soluble receptor
	Interleukin-1 converting enzyme inhibitor
Interleukin-6	Anti-interleukin-6 antibodies
	Interleukin-6 soluble receptor

fected area is called the pannus, which can have high levels of macrophages. Cartilage destruction is mediated through macrophage release of metalloproteinases such as collagenase and stromelysin, which are activated by proinflammatory cytokines, such as IL-1 and TNF-α.[16,17]

The current immune paradigm suggests that CD4 T-cells are activated following interaction with antigen presenting cells (APC) bearing MHC class II structures such as macrophages. The activated CD4 cells will then activate other cells such as macrophages, B-cells, T-cells, and synoviocytes. All of these cells have the capacity to express more cytokines, thus activating an immunological cascade. Immune activation can increase production of degenerative enzymes, and lipid metabolism.

A number of strategies have been developed to reduce the levels of unbound TNF. Since soluble receptors of TNF are found naturally occurring as cytokine sponges, various strategies have used recombinant technology to product large quantities of these products. One product is a recombinant chimeric soluble TNF receptor with a constant fragment of an immunoglobulin G.

The role of cytokines in rheumatoid arthritis is well delineated. Inflammatory mediators such as IL-1 and TNF can induce myriad biological effects. TNF is able to induce synoviocyte proliferation and enhance expression of prostaglandins, metalloproteinases, and cytokines. Inflammatory cytokines can also activate osteoclasts, thus promoting the destruction of bone tissue as well.[17]

Anticytokine therapy has utilized anti-TNF antibodies and soluble TNF receptors. Both types of strategies focus on reducing the levels of TNF for cellular binding. Reducing TNF levels correlates with a rapid improvement in joint swelling, tenderness, and morning stiffness. This further correlates to a reduction in the level of C-reactive protein, reduction of erythrocyte sedimentation rate (ESR), and reduction of blood cytokine levels. When the synovium was sent for biopsy, histological improvements paralleled with clinical manifestations.

Etanercept (Enbrel®)

Product information. Etanercept is a recombinant human TNF receptor that is linked with a constant region (Fc) of a human IgG$_1$. The hybrid protein was created by combining DNA encoding the soluble portion of human TNFR p75 and linked to DNA encoding the Fc portion. The recombinant gene was expressed in a mammalian cell line.

Pharmacology. Inflammatory cytokines such as IL-1 and TNF-α have been readily isolated from the synovial fluid of patients with rheumatoid arthritis. High levels of TNF soluble receptors (TNFSR) p55 and p75 are also present in the synovium of afflicted patients.[15,16] Soluble TNF receptors are responsible for down-regulating the activity of TNF.

In an effort to reduce TNF levels, a chimeric type II soluble TNF receptor (p75) with a constant region (Fc) of immunoglobulin G_1 (IgG_1) was tested in patients with rheumatoid arthritis. Etanercept, composed exclusively of human amino acid sequences, acts as a competitive inhibitor of TNF, thus preventing TNF binding onto TNF receptors found on the cell surface. Etanercept has been shown to block both TNF-α and TNF-β or lymphotoxin from interacting with surface receptors.[18] The inhibition of binding will reduce biologic activities mediated by TNF stimulation.[15,18] When etanercept is administered to patients with rheumatoid arthritis, it is able to reduce the concentration of proinflammatory mediators in these patients' synovium. The blockade of TNF and its mediated activity have been shown to reduce RA-related clinical events. This hybrid molecule can be used alone or in combination with methotrexate in patients who did not respond to methotrexate alone.[18]

Pharmacokinetics. Three rheumatoid arthritis patients were given a single dose of 25 mg of etanercept as a subcutaneous (SC) injection. After SC administration, the time to maximum concentration (Tmax) of etanercept was 72 hours (48 to 96 hours), where the maximum achieved concentration (Cmax) was 1.2 μg/mL (range 0.6 to 1.5 μg/mL). Median plasma half-life was determined to be 115 hours (98 to 300 hours), where drug clearance was 89 mL/h (52 mL/h per square meter).

Long-term pharmacokinetics of etanercept were studied in 25 rheumatoid arthritis patients. After six months of therapy, which consisted of 25 mg given SC twice a week, the median serum level was 3.0 μg/mL (range 1.7 to 5.6 μg/mL). No accumulation of etanercept was noted in this study, which suggested that patients may undergo a two- to fivefold increase in serum levels with repeated dosing.

Etanercept 0.4 mg/kg was given to pediatric patients with juvenile rheumatoid arthritis. Mean serum concentration was 2.1 µg/mL (0.7 to 4.3 µg/mL). No gender or age difference were seen with etanercept. Presently, there is no pharmacokinetic study evaluating patients with impaired renal or hepatic function.

Clinical trials with rheumatoid arthritis. In a randomized, multicenter, double-blinded, placebo-controlled Phase III study, patients with severe RA were treated for six months with either etanercept or placebo.[15] Etanercept, 10 mg, 25 mg, or placebo, was administered twice weekly SC. The results in the trial were expressed as percentage improvement in RA using the American College of Rheumatology (ACR) response criteria.

The results showed a statistically significant increase in 20 percent and 50 percent ACR response rates in the etanercept group. At six months, 20 percent ACR response was observed in 11, 51, and 59 percent of patients on placebo, 10 mg etanercept, and 25 mg etanercept, respectively.[15] A 50 percent ACR response was seen in 5, 24, and 40 percent of patients on placebo, 10 mg, and 25 mg, respectively.[15]

In another 24-week, randomized, double-blinded trial, 89 patients with persistently active RA despite at least six months of methotrexate therapy received either 25 mg of etanercept or placebo twice weekly while continuing methotrexate therapy.[19] As with the previous study, the primary end point in this study was a 20 percent ACR response. At the end of 24 weeks, 71 percent responded in the etanercept group, while only 27 percent achieved the same clinical outcomes in patients receiving placebo with methotrexate (p value < 0.001).[19] Further analysis showed that ACR 50 criteria was achieved in 39 percent of patients who received etanercept, when compared to only 3 percent responding in the placebo group (p value < 0.001).[19]

Clinical trials with graft rejection. Immune activation is the central obstacle in allograft rejection. This occurs when the immune system is able to recognize the transplanted graft as foreign. An immune response against the allograft is initiated by the expression of inflammatory mediators such as IL-1 and TNF.

Prevention of acute allograft rejection is the strategy of choice. However, it is impossible to totally prevent graft rejection. The onset of acute rejection will require rapid and aggressive therapy, which includes a murine anti-CD3 Mab or OKT3. Although OKT3 is effective in reducing cells that initiate graft rejection, the intense elimination of T-lymphocytes bearing CD3 surface receptors can predispose patients to infections. In addition, the administration of OKT3 can cause an infusion reaction, referred to as the OKT3 acute clinical syndrome (OKT3-ACS), which is caused by the rapid release of inflammatory mediators such as TNF and IL-1.

A number of agents have been used to reduce levels of TNF, including steroids, IL-10, and anti-TNF monoclonal antibodies.

The therapeutic potential of etanercept (TNFR:Fc), which has a higher affinity for TNF than anti-TNF, has also been studied.[20,21,22] Although patients treated with TNFR:Fc had significantly fewer symptoms from OKT3, such as chills and arthralgias, OKT3 side effects were still persistent, leading to the conclusion that OKT3-ACS is caused by multiple factors besides TNF release.

Clinical trials with septic shock. Bacteremia that leads to septic shock is related to high levels of proinflammatory mediators such as IL-1 and TNF. The elimination of either inflammatory cytokine has been suggested as a possible strategy in the treatment of septic shock.

One study[23] evaluated the role of TNF in normal healthy subjects who were given LPS. In this study, 12 subjects were given 2 ng/kg of LPS as an intravenous infusion. Thirty minutes prior to LPS administration, six patients were given etanercept (6 mg/m^2) or vehicle only.

Patients who received vehicle prior to LPS administration elicited a transient increase in plasma TNF activity, peaking after 1.5 hours (219 pg/mL; p value < 0.05). Patients that received etanercept were able to completely neutralize LPS-induced TNF activity. LPS administration was associated with an early activation of fibrinolysis (plasma concentrations of tissue-type plasminogen activator, plasminogen activator activity, and plasmin-alpha2-antiplasmin complexes), followed by inhibition (plasma plasminogen activator inhibitor type I). These changes were not observed in patients who were previously treated with etanercept, in which no LPS-induced changes in activation of coagulopathy were seen. In patients treated with etanercept, endothelial cell activation was completely ablated with a modest reduction in neutrophil activity. There was no change in the release of phospholipase A_2 or lipopolysaccharide binding protein. When etanercept was given alone without LPS, no inflammatory response was seen.[23]

The safety and efficacy of etanercept has also been evaluated in patients with septic shock.[24] In this randomized, double-blind, placebo controlled study, 141 patients were randomly assigned to receive either placebo or a single dose of etanercept at the following dosage: 0.15, 0.45, or 1.5 mg/kg. At day 28, 30 percent mortality was reported in patients receiving placebo. In the group receiving 0.1 mg/kg of etanercept, 30 percent of these patients died during the same time period. Mortality increased to 49 percent and 53 percent in the groups receiving 0.45 and 1.5 mg/kg of etanercept, which yielded a p value = 0.02 for mortality related to increased doses of etanercept. Thus, death is associated with etanercept therapy.[24]

Adverse reactions. Clinical trials reported that the most frequently encountered adverse effects associated with etanercept was injection site reactions, upper respiratory infections, and malignancies.[15,18] The injection site reactions reported in 37 percent of patients were described as mild to moderate erythema, itching, pain, or swelling. It was most frequently reported during the first month of therapy but decreased after subsequent therapy.[15,18,19]

Incidents of upper respiratory infections and sinusitis were reported in 29 percent of patients receiving etanercept versus 16 percent in the placebo group. The possibility of more serious infections exists since etanercept also blocks the immune response of TNF, a potent mediator of inflammation.[15,18,19]

A more disturbing adverse event is the development of new malignancies, which occurred in 7 out of 745 (1 percent) rheumatoid arthritis patients receiving etanercept.[18] Fortunately, this is the incidence that is expected in the population being studied.

Dosage and administration. The recommended manufactured dose is 25 mg twice weekly given as a subcutaneous injection. Continuous treatment is recommended, as symptoms have been shown to return with the discontinuation of the drug.[18] Etanercept is supplied as a sterile powder in 25 mg single-use vials and should be refrigerated at 2° to 8°C (36° to 46°F) and not frozen. The reconstituted solution should be injected immediately. However, if it is not administered immediately, it may be stored in the vial at 2° to 8°C (36° to 46°F) for up to six hours.[18]

Crohn's Disease

Autoimmune disorders such as Crohn's disease (CD) are considered inflammatory bowel diseases. This disorder is characterized by inflamed granulomatous tissue along the walls of the gastrointestinal tract.[25] Historically, mesalamine and glucocorticoids are first-line agents in the treatment of the disease. In steroid refractory Crohn's disease, immunosuppressive agents such as azathioprine, mercapto-purine, and cyclosporine are added.[26] Similar to other autoimmune diseases, CD is associated with an overexpression of several pro-inflammatory cytokines, including tumor necrosis factor-α (TNF-α), which is believed to be an important mediator of Crohn's disease.[27]

TNF-α is a cytokine produced by monocytes/macrophages and T-cells. It has been shown to induce fever, activate T-cells and granu-locytes, mediate thrombosis and fibrinolysis, aid in the development of sepsis, and lead to bone resorption, insulin resistance, and ane-mia.[28] With respect to Crohn's disease, TNF-α plays a special role in recruiting inflammatory cells to already inflamed gastrointestinal tis-sue leading to edema, activation of the coagulation cascade, and granuloma formation.[27,29] High levels of cells positive for TNF-α have been detected in the gastrointestinal mucosa in patients with Crohn's disease.[30] In fact, increased levels of TNF have been found in the feces of children with acute Crohn's, correlating strongly with disease activity.[30] Interestingly, the increased TNF-α production in Crohn's disease is localized only in the GI mucosa and lumen, com-pared to low serum levels.[27]

Many clinical trials have examined the role of TNF-α blockers in the treatment of cytokine-mediated inflammatory disorders. Among them, the TNF-α antibody, infliximab, has been shown to effectively block soluble and transmembrane TNF.[27,29]

Infliximab (Remicade®)

Product information. Infliximab is a chimeric (human/murine) Mab directed against TNF-α and is produced by a recombinant cell line cultured by continuous perfusion. Infliximab is composed of a murine Fab region that is linked to a human Fc region to prevent im-mune response against the antibody. The molecular weight of this $IgG_{1\kappa}$ is approximately 149 kDa. The affinity binding constant (Ka) is 10^{10} M^{-1} for both soluble and transmembrane TNF, preventing at-tachment to receptors.[31]

Infliximab is approved for the intravenous treatment of moderate to severe Crohn's disease refractory to other medical treatments.[31] In addition, it is also indicated for fistulizing Crohn's disease for the reduction of draining enterocutaneous fistulas. Currently, infliximab is not approved for use in the treatment of rheumatoid arthritis, although clinical trials are under way.[31]

Pharmacology. Infliximab can neutralize both soluble and transmembrane forms of TNF.[1,2,3] Infliximab does not neutralize TNF-β (lymphotoxin), a related cytokine that utilizes the same receptors as TNF-α. TNF-α has a wide range of biological activities including induction of proinflammatory cytokines such as IL-1 and IL-6, enhancement of leukocyte migration, activation of neutrophil and eosinophil functional activity, and induction of acute-phase and other liver proteins.[31] Cells expressing transmembrane TNF-α bound by infliximab can be lysed in vitro by complement or effector cells. Anti-TNF-α antibodies reduce disease activity in a cotton-toptamarin colitis model. Infliximab inhibits the functional activity of TNF-α in a wide variety of in vitro bioassays utilizing human fibroblasts, endothelial cells, neutrophils, T-lymphocytes, and epithelial cells.[31]

Pharmacokinetics. Pharmacokinetic profiles of infliximab were determined from a dose-ranging study of a single intravenous infusion of 1, 5, 10, or 20 mg/kg. These studies found that infliximab exhibits a dose-dependent increase of maximum concentration (Cmax) and AUC. An intravenous dose of 5 mg/kg infliximab resulted in a Cmax of 118 mg/mL and volume distribution of 3 L. The elimination half-life was 9.5 days.[31] Circulating levels of infliximab were detectable approximately 12 weeks after the dose, with a duration of action of 12 to 48 weeks for Crohn's disease, and 6 to 12 weeks for rheumatoid arthritis.[26,32]

Clinical trials—Crohn's disease. A randomized, double-blinded, placebo-controlled trial in patients with refractory, moderate to severe Crohn's disease studied the efficacy of a single infliximab dose compared to placebo.[29] In a dose ranging study, 13 CD patients were given a single dose of infliximab ranging from 5 to 20 mg/kg while receiving concomitant medications for Crohn's disease. Ileal and colonic biopsy specimens were collected before and four weeks after therapy and analyzed for inflammation and levels of inflammatory mediators. The results showed that both ileitis and colitis were significantly reduced in patients receiving infliximab as demonstrated by reductions in neutrophils and mononuclear cells in the GI epithelium and lamina propria. In addition, circulating levels of T-lymphocytes, interleukins, and tumor necrosis factor were sharply decreased.[29]

Another 12-week, multicenter, double-blinded, placebo-controlled trial of infliximab examined 108 patients with moderate to severe Crohn's disease resistant to other therapies.[26]

Again, patients received single doses of infliximab with dosages ranging from 5 to 20 mg/kg. The primary end point was defined as a reduction of Crohn's Disease Activity Index score of at least 70 points at four weeks. At the end of four weeks, 81 percent of the treatment group receiving 5 mg/kg achieved the primary endpoint. Fifty percent and 64 percent of the treatment groups receiving 10 mg/kg and 20 mg/kg, respectively, achieved clinical response, compared to only 17 percent of the placebo group. In addition, 33 percent of the treatment group achieved complete remission of disease (score below 150 in activity index), compared to only 4 percent of placebo patients. At 12 weeks, 41 percent of the treatment group had reached the primary end point.[26]

Another multicenter, randomized, placebo-controlled trial of 94 patients with fistulizing disease compared infliximab with placebo.[33] Treatment patients received either 5 or 10 mg/kg infliximab at zero, two, and six weeks. Concurrent therapy was kept stable for both groups during the trial. The primary end point was a greater than 50 percent reduction of open fistulae on two consecutive visits. Results showed that 68 percent of the 5 mg/kg treatment group achieved ≥ 50 percent reduction in the number of draining fistulas, compared to 26 percent of the placebo group. Fifty-five percent of the treatment group achieved complete closure of all fistulas, compared to 13 percent of the placebo group.[33]

Dosage and administration. The recommended dose for active Crohn's disease is one dose of 5 mg/kg given intravenously over at least two hours. For fistulizing disease, the dose is 5 mg/kg once, then repeat at two and six weeks after the first infusion. For rheumatoid arthritis, the recommended dose is 10 mg/kg one time only.[31] Infliximab is available as a sterile powder in single-dose, 100 mg vials and should be stored between 2° to 8°C (36° to 46°F) and not frozen.[31]

Adverse reactions. The most common adverse reaction reported with the use of infliximab is nausea. Other reactions include headache, upper respiratory infections, fatigue, chest pain, and myalgia. All reactions were reported to be similar to placebo.[26,31] It is also worth noting that patients who were re-treated with infliximab, after intervals of two to four years, experienced serum-sickness type reactions three to 12 days after the infusion.[31] Because infliximab is a chimeric antibody, the potential does exist for immune reactions when patients are retreated with the drug.

TNF-α SOLUBLE RECEPTOR p55-IgG₁ FUSION PROTEIN

One of the anticytokine therapies evaluated for use in sepsis patients was $p55\text{-}IgG_1$. This recombinant chimeric protein contains both type I TNF receptor and immunoglobulin G_1 sequences ($p55\text{-}IgG_1$). One randomized, double-blind, placebo-controlled study, where 498 patients were stratified to receive a single infusion of $p55\text{-}IgG_1$ at 0.083 mg/kg, 0.042 mg/kg, or 0.008 mg/kg, was compared to patients receiving placebo.

A low dose of p55-IgG (0.042 mg/kg) was able to reduce mortality by 5 percent at day 28 of therapy. When higher doses (0.083 mg/kg) were administered, a 15 percent reduction in mortality at day 28 was realized. Despite a trend toward reduction of mortality, the difference between the group receiving active drug and placebo was not statistically significant. However, there was a significant reduction in mortality when predicted mortality and plasma IL-6 levels were included in the regression analysis.

NOTES

1. Arend WP, Dayer JM. Inhibition of the production and effects of interleukin-1 and tumor necrosis factor alpha in rheumatoid arthritis [Review] [101 refs]. *Arthritis & Rheumatism* 1995;38(2):151-160.

2. Arend WP, Leung DY. IgG induction of IL-1 receptor antagonist production by human monocytes. *Immunological Reviews* 1994;139:71-78.

3. Arend WP. Interleukin-1 receptor antagonist. A new member of the interleukin-1 family. *Journal of Clinical Investigation* 1991;88(5):1445-1451.

4. Fischer E, Van Zee KJ, Marano MA, Rock CS, Kenney JS, Poutsiaka DD, Dinarello CA, Lowry SF, Moldawer LL. Interleukin-1 receptor antagonist circulates in experimental inflammation and in human disease. *Blood* 1992;79(9):2196-2200.

5. Dinarello CA, Thompson RC. Blocking IL-1: Interleukin-1 receptor antagonist in vivo and in vitro [Review] [84 refs]. *Immunology Today* 1991;12(11):404-410.

158   HANDBOOK OF PHARMACEUTICAL BIOTECHNOLOGY

6. Dinarello CA, Wolff SM. The role of interleukin-1 in disease [published erratum appears in *New England Journal of Medicine* 1993;328(10):744] [Review] [51 refs]. *New England Journal of Medicine* 1993;328(2):106-113.

7. Ohlsson K, Bjork P, Bergenfeldt M, Hageman R, Thompson RC. Interleukin-1 receptor antagonist reduces mortality from endotoxin shock. *Nature* 1990; 348(6301):550-552.

8. Everaerdt B, Brouckaert P, Fiers W. Recombinant IL-1 receptor antagonist protects against TNF-induced lethality in mice. *Journal of Immunology* 1994; 152(10):5041-5049.

9. Ferretti M, Casini-Raggi V, Pizarro TT, Eisenberg SP, Nast CC, Cominelli F. Neutralization of endogenous IL-1 receptor antagonist exacerbates and prolongs inflammation in rabbit immune colitis [see comments]. *Journal of Clinical Investigation* 1994;94(1):449-453.

10. Casini-Raggi V, Kam L, Chong YJ, Fiocchi C, Pizarro TT, Cominelli F. Mucosal imbalance of IL-1 and IL-1 receptor antagonist in inflammatory bowel disease. A novel mechanism of chronic intestinal inflammation. *Journal of Immunology* 1995;154(5):2434-2440.

11. Granowitz EV, Porat R, Mier JW, Pribble JP, Stiles DM, Bloedow DC, Catalano MA, Wolff SM, Dinarello CA. Pharmacokinetics, safety and immunomodulatory effects of human recombinant interleukin-1 receptor antagonist in healthy humans. *Cytokine* 1992;4(5):353-360.

12. Fisher C, Agosti JM, Opal SM, Lowry SF, Balk RA, Sadoff JC, Abraham E, Schein RM, Benjamin E. Treatment of septic shock with the tumor necrosis factor receptor: Fc fusion protein. The Soluble TNF Receptor Sepsis Study Group. *New England Journal of Medicine* 1996;334(26):1697-1702.

13. Shen WC, Louie SG. *Immunology for pharmacists and pharmaceutical scientists.* Singapore: Harwood Press, 1998.

14. Dinarello CA. Interleukin-1 and interleukin-1 antagonism [Review] [326 refs]. *Blood* 1991;77(8):1627-1652.

15. Moreland LW, Schiff MH, Baumgartner SW. Etanercept therapy in rheumatoid arthritis: A randomized, controlled trial. *Annal of Internal Medicine* 1999; 130:478-486.

16. Feldman M, Brennan FM, Maini RN. Role of cytokines in rheumatoid arthritis. *Annual Reviews of Immunology* 1996;14:397-440.

17. Harris ED Jr. Etiology and pathogenesis of rheumatoid arthritis. *Textbook of rheumatology,* Fourth edition. Philadelphia, PA: WB Saunders Company, 1993, pp. 833-873.

18. Product Information: Enbrel™, etanercept. Wyeth-Ayerst Laboratories and Immunex, Seattle, WA, 1998.

19. Weinblatt ME, Kremer JM, Bankhurst AD. A trial of etanercept, a recombinant tumor necrosis factor receptor: Fc fusion protein, in patients with rheumatoid arthritis receiving methotrexate. *New England Journal of Medicine* 1999;340(4): 253-259.

20. Novak EJ, Blosch CM, Perkins J, Davis CL, Barr D, McVicar JP, Griffin RS, Farrand AL, Wener M, Marsh C. Recombinant human tumor necrosis factor receptor Fc fusion protein therapy in kidney transplant recipients undergoing OKT3 induction therapy. *Transplantation* 1998;66(12):1732-1735.

21. Easton JD, Pascual M, Wee S, Farrell M, Phelan J, Boskovic S, Blosch C, Mohler KM, Cosimi AB. Evaluation of recombinant human soluble dimeric tumor necrosis factor receptor for prevention of OKT3-associated acute clinical syndrome. *Transplantation* 1996;61(2):224-228.

22. Wee S, Pascual M, Eason JD, Schoenfeld DA, Phelan J, Boskovic S, Blosch C, Mohler K, Cosimi AB. Biological effects and fate of a soluble, dimeric, 80-kDa tumor necrosis factor receptor in renal transplant recipients who receive OKT3 therapy. *Transplantation* 1997;63(4):570-577.

23. Rogy MA, Coyle SM, Oldenburg HS, Rock CS, Barie PS, Van Zee KJ, Smith CG, Moldawer LL, Lowry SF. Persistently elevated soluble tumor necrosis factor receptor and interleukin-1 receptor antagonist levels in critically ill patients. *Journal of the American College of Surgeons* 1994;178(2):132-138.

24. Fisher CJ Jr., Agosti JM, Opal SM, Lowry SF, Balk RA, Sadoff JC, Abraham E, Schein RM, Benjamin E. Treatment of septic shock with the tumor necrosis factor receptor: Fc fusion protein. The Soluble TNF Receptor Sepsis Study Group. *New England Journal of Medicine* 1996;334(26):1697-1702.

25. Levine DS. Clinical features and complications of Crohn's disease. In Targan S, Shanahan F, eds. *Inflammatory bowel disease: From bench to bedside*. Baltimore: Williams and Wilkins, 1993, pp. 296-316.

26. Targan SR, Hanauer SB, Deventer SJ, Mayer L, Present DH, Braakman T, DeWoody KL, Schiable TF, Rutgeerts PJ. A short-term study of chimeric monoclonal antibody cA2 to tumor necrosis factor-α for Crohn's disease. *New England Journal of Medicine* 1997;337:1029-1035.

27. Deventer SJV. Tumor necrosis factor and Crohn's disease. *Gut* 1997;40:443-448.

28. Tracey KJ, Cerami A. Tumor necrosis factor: A pleiotropic cytokine and therapeutic agent. *Annual Review of Medicine* 1994;45:491-503.

29. Baert FJ, D'Haens GR, Peeters M, Hiele MI, Schiable TF, Shealy D, Geboes K, Rutgeerts PJ. Tumor necrosis factor alpha antibody (infliximab) therapy profoundly down-regulates the inflammation in Crohn's ileocolitis. *Gastroenterology* 1999;116:22-28.

30. Braegger CP, Nichols S, Murch SH, Stephens S, MacDonald TT. Tumor necrosis factor alpha in stool as a marker for intestinal inflammation. *Lancet* 1992;339:89-91.

31. Product Information: Remicade, Infliximab. Centocor, Malvern, PA, 1998.

32. Elliot MJ, Maini RN, Feldmann M, Long-Fox A, Charles P, Bijl H, Woody JN. Repeated therapy with monoclonal antibody to tumor necrosis factor alpha (cA2) in patients with rheumatoid arthritis. *Lancet* 1994;344(8930):1125-1127.

33. Present D, Mayer L, Deventer SJ. Anti-TNF-alpha chimeric antibody (cA2) is effective in the treatment of the fistulae of Crohn's disease. *American Journal of Gastroenterology* 1997;92:1746.

Chapter 7

Oligonucleotide and Gene Therapy

Stan G. Louie
Amir Aminimanizani
Parul Patel

INTRODUCTION

Gene therapy is essentially the introduction of a normally functioning gene, known as wild type (WT), into a target cell. Since the late 1980s, gene therapy treatments have fast become the theoretical hope as a cure for various diseases. The technology behind gene therapy has come to fruition, and ongoing clinical trials continue to assess its safety and efficacy.

Enthusiasm for gene therapy has been fueled by evidence suggesting that normal function can be restored when a WT gene is inserted into a cell carrying a dysfunctional version of that gene. Various diseases have been identified as disorders in which the pathogenesis is either a gene deficiency or genetic mutation (Table 7.1). The insertion of WT genes into target cells found in these individuals may ameliorate symptoms of the disease or even provide a cure. Gene deficiency syndromes, such as adenosine deaminase (ADA) deficiency, β-thalassemia, cystic fibrosis (CF), and Gaucher's disease, are areas in which gene therapy is being tested. One important factor determining the success of gene replacement is that adequate concentrations of the gene product are produced.

In contrast, some disorders are caused by an overproduction of the gene products, thus potential therapeutic agents may block the effects of the causative gene. Blockade of gene expression could be accomplished by inserting a stop codon or "nonsense" sequence into the internal domains of that specific gene. This technology can also be used

TABLE 7.1. Genetic Disorders with Possible Gene Therapy Candidates

Genetic Disorders	Target Gene Delivery
Adenosine deaminase deficiency	Adenosine deaminase (ADA)
β-thalasemia	Hemoglobin
	β-globulin
Cystic fibrosis	Cystic fibrosis transmembrane conductance receptor (CFTR)
Cancers	p53 tumor suppressor gene
	Multiple drug resistance (MDR)
	Dihydrofolate reductase (DHFR)
Brain tumors	Thymidine kinase (TK)
Gaucher's disease	β-Glucocerebrodidase

to terminate genes that have been linked to tumorigenesis, such as the oncogenes *c-myc, erb-2, HER-2,* and *ras.*

OLIGONUCLEOTIDE THERAPY

Oligonucleotide therapy is another strategy that is used in gene therapy. The goal of oligonucleotide therapy is to selectively inhibit mRNA translation to specific proteins that may lead to undesirable biological activities. Oligonucleotides or antisense oligonucleotides are short segments of complementary RNA that can hybridize to a segment of target mRNA through hydrogen bonding. Upon reaching the target mRNA in either the cytoplasm or nucleus, the oligonucleotide will bind and form a double-stranded RNA segment. This formation is recognized by the enzyme RNAse H, which then cleaves the target mRNA releasing the oligonucleotide to hybridize another target mRNA for the process to repeat. Elimination of mRNA will inhibit protein synthesis.

To be therapeutically beneficial, the oligonucleotide must be of a certain length. The optimal length varies depending on a number of factors, including the type of expression vector, but typically consists of 12 to 20 nucleotides, thus lending to the term *oligomer.* If the oligomer is too long, cellular enzymes quickly degrade it. In addition, longer oligomers are more difficult to deliver into cells. However, shorter oligomers have problems hybridizing to target mRNA, thus decreasing their effectiveness.[1] The optimal oligomer length is dependent on the biological temperature, pH of the environment, secondary and tertiary structures, and number of G-C base pairs found in the target sequence.[2] Once these and other factors have been investigated experimentally, the oligonucleotide is constructed via an automated DNA synthesizer.

The synthesized oligonucleotide is usually modified in order to increase its resistance to nucleases, such as DNAse, that degrade phosphodiester linkages. Modifications may include replacing the phosphodiester backbone with a phosphorothioate, altering the ribose moiety, and attaching the oligonucleotide to DNA-protein complexes or cationic liposomes.[3] However, with any type of modification, the oligonucleotide must retain its binding capacity, affinity for target sequences, and ability to internalize cells.

To combat the problem of cell penetration, carrier systems have been designed to protect the oligonucleotide and enhance cell delivery. Oligomers have been incorporated into the bilayers of spherical phospholipid membranes called liposomes. At the target site, the oligomer can partition out of the liposome for activity. In fact, the oligomer-liposome can have targeting ability if monoclonal antibodies are attached to the complex.[1] Other approaches to enhance oligonucleotide delivery include attachment to poly-L-lysine water-soluble polymeric carriers and adsorption onto nanoparticles.[1]

Despite these improvements, antisense therapy has problems that include a short in vivo half-life, a large dose requirement for efficacy, parenteral administration, and the need for sophisticated cell targeting moieties.[3] Oligonucleotide therapy has been investigated in the treatment of hypertension with antisense oligonucleotides to angiotensinogen, and in leukemia with oligonucleotides against bone marrow progenitor cells of leukemia.[3]

Fomivirsen (Vitravene®)

Human cytomegalovirus (CMV) is a ubiquitous organism, which is the cause of severe morbidity and mortality in immunocompromised patients. CMV retinitis emerged in the early 1980s as a common opportunistic infection in patients with AIDS.[4,5] Prior to the introduction of protease inhibitors, the incidence of CMV retinitis was approximately 21 to 44 percent in HIV patients with CD4+ counts < 50 cells/mm.[6] Without therapy, CMV will rapidly progress causing CMV-mediated blindness and spreading into other visceral organs.

Prior to the introduction of fomivirsen, all anti-CMV agents had similar mechanisms of action, namely inhibiting viral polymerase. Ganciclovir, foscarnet, and cidofovir inhibit the activity of the CMV DNA polymerase, which is essential for viral replication.[5] There are several limitations to the use of these therapies. These anti-CMV drugs are virustatic, which means they only slow the progression of disease.[7] Since these agents are virustatic, the emergence of resistance occurs in about 10 percent of previously treated patients. Resistant viruses will have reduced sensitivity to DNA polymerase inhibitors.[7] More important, anti-CMV agents are associated with adverse effects such as nephrotoxicity and bone marrow suppression.[4,5,7]

The development of newer, more effective anti-CMV therapies is essential for the treatment of CMV. Antisense therapy is a new therapeutic approach that utilizes synthetic oligonucleotides to inhibit a wide variety of viruses including herpes simplex, influenza, papilloma, and CMV.[4,8] Antisense oligonucleotides are short nucleotide sequences that bind onto specific mRNA sequences.[4,7]

Product Information

Fomivirsen is an antisense oligonucleotide that is injected directly into the eye for the treatment of CMV retinitis. Unlike other pharmaceutical agents, antisense oligonucleotides are a mirror image of the natural RNA strand or sense sequence, and will bind tightly on complement sense sequence.

Pharmacology

Fomivirsen is a phosphorothioate oligonucleotide that binds onto viral mRNA sequences encoding for immediate early region 2 (IE2). IE2 encodes several proteins responsible for regulation of viral gene expression. The binding of fomivirsen onto IE2 mRNA sequences will activate RNAse H, an enzyme that cleaves the viral mRNA sequence, thus inhibiting further protein synthesis. Inhibition of vital protein synthesis can inhibit production of infectious CMV.

Pharmacokinetics

Following an intravitreal injection, fomivirsen is cleared from the vitreous over the course of seven to ten days. The highest concentrations of fomivirsen are found in the retina and iris, where concentrations initially increased over the first three to five days. A steady decline of fomivirsen is observed over time. The mechanism of antisense clearance from the eye is a combination of tissue distribution and metabolism. Metabolism in the eye is the primary route of elimination for fomivirsen. It is metabolized by endonucleases in a process that sequentially removes residues from the terminal ends of the oligonucleotide yielding shortened oligonucleotides and mononucleotide metabolites. Mononucleotides are further catabolized to endogenous nucleotides and are excreted as low molecular weight metabolites.[7]

Systemic exposure to fomivirsen following single or repeated intravitreal injections in animal studies revealed that nearly undetectable levels of antisense are found in the blood. Fomivirsen is minimally absorbed into systemic circulation.[7] In monkeys treated every other week for up to three months with fomivirsen, metabolites of the parent antisense molecula were found in liver, kidney, and plasma at detectable levels.[7]

Clinical Trials

Few published clinical trials in human subjects are available for assessing the efficacy and safety of fomivirsen. In one such trial, 54 patients with previously treated CMV retinitis were assigned to two separate treatment groups. One group received fomvirisen (330 µg) once a week, given as an intravitreal injection, for three weeks, that is followed by an injection every two weeks for maintenance. The second group received 330 µg of fomivirsen on days 1 and 15, then every four weeks during maintenance. The results of the second group showed a median time to CMV retinitis progression of 267 days.[7] This was as good as outcomes from ganciclovir therapy.

Another trial compared the in vitro effects of fomivirsen with ganciclovir on human dermal fibroblasts. Fomivirsen was found to be at least 30 times more potent than ganciclovir.[4] The EC_{50} of the antisense drug was 0.1 µM, compared to an EC_{50} of 3 µM for ganciclovir. Both fomivirsen and ganciclovir reduced viral replication by two log units at concentrations of 2.2 and 38 μM, respectively, suggesting that these agents have comparable potency with standard of care.[4]

Dosage and Administration

Fomivirsen is manufactured in a single-use vial containing 6.6 mg/mL for intravitreal injection only.[7] The recommended induction dose of fomivirsen for CMV retinitis is 330 μg given as an intravitreal injection every other week for two doses. This is followed by maintenance therapy, which consists of 330 μg by intravitreal injection every four weeks.[7] The drug is administered by intravitreal injection (0.05 mL/eye) using a 30-gauge needle-fitted tuberculin syringe. If not used immediately, fomivirsen should be stored between 2° and 25°C (35° to 77°F) and protected from excessive heat and light.[7]

Adverse Reactions

The most commonly observed adverse reaction is ocular inflammation, including iritis and vitritis, usually during the induction phase of therapy. Limited published data from human and animal studies indicate that approximately 5 to 20 percent of subjects experienced blurred vision, eye pain, photophobia, increased intraocular pressure, fever, headache, sinusitis, and vomiting.[7] Ocular inflammation can be managed by application of topical corticosteroids. Intraocular pressure (IOP) should be monitored with each visit and should be treated with drugs that lower IOP.[7]

ras-*ANTISENSE THERAPY*

Dysregulation of various genes has been associated with various oncogenic processes. One family of genes that has been linked to oncogenesis is the *ras* oncogene family. *ras* oncogenes have been found in animal viruses, such as Harvey murine sarcoma viral gene (H-*ras*) and Kirsten murine sarcoma viral gene (K-*ras*). The oncogenic nature of *ras* has been demonstrated: when the protein for *ras* is overproduced, the transfected cells seem to develop neoplastic characteristics.

The *ras* gene encodes for a protein with a molecular weight of 21 kDa and is more commonly referred to as p21. p21 is an enzyme that is found primarily on the inner surfaces of the plasma membrane. Guanosine triphosphate (GTP) binds onto p21, which is responsible for activation and subsequent intracellular signal transduction. The ultimate consequence of GTP-dependent activation usually results in transcription of other regulatory proteins. Along with intracellular activation, p21 is also responsible for termination of signal transduction. Here, p21 serves as an "on or off" switch. The termination of the intracellular signal, which is also known as an "off" signal, often occurs when GTP is hydrolyzed to yield inorganic phosphate and guanosine 5'-diphosphate (GDP). p21 regulation may be disrupted if an alteration of the *ras* gene occurs, which may lead to oncogenesis. In this scenario, *ras* activates the intracellular signals.

On this basis, a strategy for gene therapy involving the inactivation of oncogenes has been developed using gene constructs that express antisense RNA and ribozymes. Antisense RNA and ribozymes are oligonucleotide-based therapies that consist of complementary bases which bind onto the target mRNA, thus blocking transcription. Both antisense and ribozymes bind onto target mRNA, thereby eliminating mRNA splicing, transport, transcription, or translation. Unlike antisense RNA, ribozymes have inherent catalytic activity for cleaving the phosphodiester bonds in target RNA. In contrast, antisense binds onto an mRNA portion, thus inhibiting protein assembly. Prolonged binding onto mRNA will initiate RNAse H, which will degrade the complex.

One study showed that the expression of retroviral K-*ras* antisense RNA gene in lung cancer led to a substantial (90 percent) decrease in K-*ras* protein transcription, and a tenfold suppression of cancer cell proliferation.[9] Likewise, another study utilizing the adenoviral anti-H-*ras* ribozyme gene showed a significant decrease in H-*ras* transcription, which correlated with the suppression of tumor proliferation.[10]

These promising results have become the impetus of various antisense agents, such as therapy for cancer using *raf,* intracelullar adhesion molecule, and vascular adhesion molecule as targets. Antisense therapy is also being investigated for the treatment of viral infections such as HIV, HCV, and human papilloma virus.

GENE DELIVERY SYSTEMS

For gene therapy to be successful, the delivery of the desired gene is crucial. A number of methods have been developed to deliver the desired genes into targeted cells. These techniques include microinjection, electroporation, liposomes, and viral vectors (Table 7.2). Microinjection is the direct placement of genetic material into the nucleus, whereas electroporation utilizes an electric charge that will increase cellular membrane permeability, allowing the delivery of recombinant DNA vectors (Figure 7.1). Recombinant DNA can also be incorporated into artificial lipid vesicles, called liposomes. Encapsulated genes can attach to the targeted cells and fuse with cellular membranes, thus delivering the gene intracellularly. One advantage of using liposomal delivery systems is the ability to circumvent the endocytic vesicles that degrade genetic material.

The use of viruses as gene delivery vehicles has also been employed. Viral-mediated gene delivery involves the construction of recombinant viral particles that will transfer novel genes into cells by the process of infection. The main objective of viral-mediated gene transfer is to take advantage of highly evolved processes that enable viruses to transfect cells by inserting their own genetic material into host cells. Oftentimes, viral genes can incorporate or integrate into the host cell genome.

TABLE 7.2. Delivery Systems for Gene Therapy

System	Technique/Vector
Nonviral delivery system	DNA complexation
	Microinjection
	Electroporation
	Liposomes
Viral delivery system	Adenovirus
	Parvovirus/adeno-associated virus (AAV)
	Retrovirus
	Herpesvirus
	Vaccinia virus

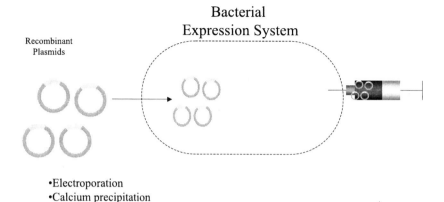

•Electroporation
•Calcium precipitation

FIGURE 7.1. Methods of delivering recombinant genes

Several different virus systems have been used as potential vehicles: adenovirus, adeno-associated virus (AAV), herpes virus, vaccinia virus, poliovirus, and retroviruses. Each of these vehicles has its own advantages and disadvantages, which are reviewed in Table 7.3. Transfection using recombinant DNA-carrying viruses is not very complicated. First, viral particles are harvested from the supernatant of infected cells. Next, the DNA is extracted and coprecipitated using calcium chloride. The precipitated DNA complex is then added to uninfected target cells. After an incubation period, infectious viral particles can be found in the supernatant of the transfected cells, which are excellent gene carriers because retroviruses do not induce lysis of the host cell as is common in other virus vector systems.

Other advantages associated with using retroviruses include the ability to infect a wide variety of target cells. A unique characteristic of retroviruses is that they use RNA as their genetic template. In order to convert an RNA template into DNA codes, retroviruses use an enzyme called reverse transcriptase that catalyzes the conversion into complementary DNA (cDNA) codes. Retroviruses are efficient in integrating the viral genome into the host cell genome, serving as a provirus template for protein synthesis in the formation of new viral particles.

TABLE 7.3. Comparison of Viral Vectors

Characteristic	Retrovirus	Adenovirus	HSV	AAV
Insert size	8 kb	7-8 kb	30 kb	4.5 kb
Insert site	Genome (random)	Nucleus	Cytoplasm	Chromosome 19
Require host replication	Yes	No	No	No
Gene expression	Stable (>1 year)	Transient (2-4 weeks)	Poor	Stable?
Replication competent	No	Yes/no	Yes/no	No
Transduction efficiency	Variable	High	Low	High
Oncogenicity	Yes	Yes	?	?
Titer (log)	6-7	11-12	8	4
In vivo delivery	Poor	High	High	High
Tropism	Neuron, T-cell	Respiratory epithelium	Neuron	?
Target cells	• Fibroblast • Myeloblast • Smooth muscle • Hematopoietic cells	• Hepatocyte • Airway epithelial • Lymphoid • Hematopoietic cells	• Neuron • Hepatocytes	• Fibroblast • Hematopoietic cells
Advantages	• Integration into host genome • Stable expression • Vector protein not expressed in host	• High viral titers • Infect dividing & nondividing cells	• Large insert size • High viral titers • Infect dividing and nondividing cells • No integration (safe)	• Cause no known human disease • Infect dividing & nondividing cells • Crosses blood-brain barrier (BBB)
Disadvantages	• Random integration • Infect only dividing cells • Low viral titers • Immunogenicity • Poor in vivo delivery	• Transient expression • Potential to recombine with wild type	• Transient expression • Potential to recombine with wild type	• Requires adenovirus as helper virus low transduction • Efficiency may be cytotoxic helper • Virus may be Low transduction low viral titers Small • Insert size integration

One of the problems associated with using viruses is that viral infection can potentially kill the host cell. In addition, viruses can alter growth properties of the infected cells, and thus may lead to tumorigenesis. Most viral vectors are unable to multiply and cause pathogenicity in the host through natural recombination with another virus. Despite using nonreplicating vehicles, viruses may reacquire pathogenicity through recombination with other viruses.

Viral Vectors

Depending on the gene of interest, different types of vectors may be selected for the application of gene therapy. A summary of selected viral vectors, their characteristics, target cells, and advantages and disadvantages associated with each system is presented in Table 7.3.

Retrovirus

Retroviruses infect only dividing cells, thus making them a useful tool in the gene therapy of glioma cells. This gene delivery system targets rapidly dividing tumor cells found in the brain. More important, retroviral vectors cannot infect normal nondividing brain cells. Since a retrovirus can integrate into the host genome, it is the vector of choice when permanent expression of a foreign gene is necessary. For example, retroviral vectors can be used to transfer cytokine genes as a means of vaccination.

Unfortunately, retroviral vectors also have disadvantages such as random viral insertion into the host genome, which can lead to mutational oncogenesis. Furthermore, the capacity of gene transfer (8 kb) and viral titer (10^7 pfu/mL) is quite low as compared to other vectors.

Adenovirus

Adenovirus is preferred over retrovirus if stable expression is not necessary because viral genes reside as an episomal vector in the nucleus of the cell and do not integrate into the genome. As the adenoviral vectors undergo cellular degradation, gene expression can be easily lost. This transient level of gene expression also means that it has a lower oncogenic potential than the retrovirus vector. One potential use of adenoviral vectors in cancer therapy is the delivery of virally directed prodrug gene therapy, such as the herpes simplex virus thymidine kinase *(HSV-tk)* gene, in which the gene needs to be expressed only long enough to sensitize the tumor for chemotherapy. Following the introduction of gene into tumor cells, cells containing the new gene are eliminated by antiviral agents since these genes render the cells sensitive to these agents.

Unlike retroviruses, high viral titers can be easily achieved ($10^{11\text{-}12}$ plaque-forming units [PFU]/mL). Another advantage of adenovirus is its capability of infecting slowly dividing cells, such as cells of the respiratory system and liver. In fact, adeno-associated viruses (AAV) have a high tropism for lung epithelial, which led to one of the earliest successful trials with gene therapy in cystic fibrosis. In this study, the cystic fibrosis transmembrane conduction reductase gene (CFTR) was inserted into lung epithelia using nebulized vectors.[11] Unfortunately, it was discovered that adenoviral vectors are able to elicit an undesirable immune response, thus repeated administration of adenoviral vectors is prohibited. Another potential problem associated with using adenovirus is that the vector may regain replication competency. This occurs when the virus is able to reacquire the ability to replicate through homologous recombination with the wild-type adenovirus found in the body.

Herpes Simplex Virus and Adeno-Associated Virus

Herpes simplex virus (HSV) offers the major advantage of a large gene (30 kb) transfer capacity. In particular, the tropism for neuronal cells and the ability to penetrate the blood-brain barrier renders it the vector of choice for treating brain tumors.[12] Adeno-associated virus (AAV) requires a helper virus such as adenovirus, to supply the essential genes for viral production. Therefore, it has a low potential of inducing oncogenicity and immunogenicity. However, as with other viruses, the risk of reacquiring virulence through the contamination with a helper virus or wild-type AAV is always possible. Similar to adenovirus, AAV vectors are usually unable to specifically integrate into chromosomes.[13] However, unlike adenovirus, AAV titers are substantially lower than other viral vectors (10^4 PFU/mL), a major disadvantage for use.

Nonviral Vectors

Nonviral vectors do not have the potential to cause disease and are less immunogenic than viral vectors. Table 7.4 summarizes the properties of selected nonviral vectors. In general, nonviral vectors can ac-

TABLE 7.4. Comparison of Nonviral Vectors

Characteristic	Plasmid DNA Injection	Liposome	Ballistic DNA Injection	Receptor-DNA-Mediated Transfer
Insert size	>20 kb	>20 kb	>20 kb	>20 kb
Insertion site	Cytoplasm	Cytoplasm	Cytoplasm	Cytoplasm
Require host replication	No	No	No	No
Gene expression	Transient	Transient	Transient	Transient
Replication competent	No	No	No	No
In vivo delivery	Poor	Variable	Exposed tissues	Poor
Advantages	• Large insert size • Nontoxic	• Large insert size • Low toxic potential	• Large insert size • Low toxic potential • Do not cause disease	• Large insert size • Cell-specific targeting
Useful for vaccination	• Immunogenicity • Do not cause disease	• Immunogenicity • Do not cause disease	• Do not cause disease	
Disadvantages	• Inefficient gene transfer • Unstable gene transfer	• Less efficient gene transfer than viruses • Unstable gene	• Inefficient and unstable gene transfer • Requires surgical procedure	• Low in vivo gene expression

commodate a much larger gene capacity (> 20 kb) than can viral vectors. Nevertheless, gene delivery through nonviral vectors is usually inefficient and unstable relative to viral vectors.

One method of nonviral gene transfer is the direct injection of naked plasmid DNA into the muscles. Direct DNA injection is a simple, cheap, and nontoxic procedure relative to viral delivery. However, it can be used only to deliver genes into skin, thymus, and muscle tissues. A study injecting DNA into mouse skeletal muscle showed significant levels of gene expression of the reporter gene.[14] Unfortunately, only a low percentage of myofibers express the genes following a single injection. Since the DNA exists as an unstable episome, in vivo expression is transient. However, this technology can be utilized in the production of DNA vaccines in which continual protein synthesis is not required for activity.

Ballistic DNA injection, also known as particle bombardment, microprojectile gene transfer, or the "gene-gun," is another nonviral delivery method. This method involves coating plasmid DNA onto the surface of 1 to 3 micron diameter gold or tungsten beads. Using an electric discharge device or gas pulse, these particles are accelerated and fired at the tissue through the membrane barrier. This method is more complicated than using viral vectors requiring surgical procedures and in vivo delivery is limited to exposed tissues. Furthermore, physical manipulation of the target cell may also cause cell death.

Liposomes

Liposomes can be used as nonviral vectors for gene delivery. The preparation of a liposomal DNA complex is relatively simple in comparison with viral vector preparations. Liposomes are formed by exploiting the interactions between amphilic compounds and the aqueous medium in which they are resuspended. There are various methods of producing the type and size of liposomes. The types of liposomes produced are dependent on (1) the composition of the vesicles, (2) how the dried constituents are rehydrated, and (3) the properties of the reconstitution solution. Another factor influencing the size and type of liposome formed includes the hydration process in which the lipid emulsion is agitated by various means (sonication, French pressure).

The size and character of liposomes are predominately determined by the constituents. The components constituting the lipid bilayers will also determine the shelf life and potential toxicities associated with liposomal administration. The most important components are the amphilic phospholipids which have both hydrophobic and hydrophilic characters. Phospholipid components have two hydrophobic acyl fatty acid chains and a hydrophilic polar head. Other important constituents include cholesterol molecules, which are a major component in natural membranes.

Cholesterol is an amphipathic molecule; however, it does not form bilayer structure. Rather the concentration of cholesterol can influence the liquidlike or fluid nature of these lipid complexes. This is accomplished through interaction of the rigid steroid molecule with the acyl chains, thus restricting the acyl chains' freedom of motion in the bilayer. The addition of cholesterol can both increase and decrease the fluidity of the bilayer that is dependent on the composition of the vesicles.

Liposomes using unsaturated phospholipids usually consist of phosphtidylcholine (PC), phosphatidic acid (PA), and phoshotidylglycerol (PG). Saturated phospholipids usually include dimyristoyl phosphatidylglycerol (DMPG), dimyristoyl phoshatidylcholine (DMPC), dipalmitoyl phoshatididic acid (DPPA), and dipalmitoyl phoshatidylcholine (DPPC). When charged vesicles are desired, stearylamine is often used for positively charged liposomes, whereas cholesterol is used to stabilize lipid bilayers.

After the components for vesicle formation have been chosen, the lipids are dissolved in volatile organic solvents, such as chloroform, diethyl ether, ethanol, or the combination of any of these solvents. The phospholipids are then coated onto the walls of the container via evaporation of the organic reagents. The formation of lipid bilayers is initiated by the rehydration of the lipids coated on the walls of the container. Aqueous solution, such as buffers and salt solution, will create an environment in which hydrophobic lipids will form aggregates and the hydrophilic heads will be exposed to the aqueous medium. The hydrophobic lipid tails will aggregate and form hydrogen bonds to give rise to lipid bilayers. In the process of forming lipid bilayers, the aqueous medium will be trapped within the lipid complexes.

The percentage of aqueous solution entrapment is dependent on the time of exposure and the conditions by which the mixture is agitated. A shorter hydration period with vigorous agitation produces vesicles with low entrapment efficiency. In contrast, when the same lipid constituents are allowed to hydrate for a longer period with gentle agitation, their entrapment capacity will increase. Entrapment efficiency can also be influenced by the thickness of the lipid film and the amount of aqueous solution that is entrapped. Thinner lipid film has been associated with increased entrapment capacity.

Cationic liposomes have the ability to form stable complexes with the negatively charged DNA phosphate backbone. The lipid portion of the liposome adsorbs into the cell membrane and delivers the associated nucleic acid into the cytoplasm. The liposome itself can protect the DNA from cellular degradative processes for a certain amount of time. Furthermore, liposomes can be degraded by biological enzymes.

CURRENT STRATEGIES FOR CANCER GENE THERAPY

Strategies to introduce therapeutic genes for the treatment of cancer have been rapidly progressing. In general, these strategies can be categorized into two classes, namely, the insertion of inhibitory genes, and/or the insertion of functional or "wild-type" genes that restore gene function. Examples of inhibitory oligonucleotide therapies are the insertion of an RNA antisense oligonucleotide or ribozyme gene. Alternatively, the insertion of a wild-type tumor suppressor gene can block the overexpression of oncogenes such as *c-myc* and *ras*.

Another strategy in the treatment against cancer is to stimulate the immune system. This can be accomplished by inserting a stimulatory cytokine gene into malignant tissues. The expression of this stimulatory cytokine will prime the immune system to localize at the site of cytokine secretion (tumor tissue), and activate host defense to eliminate any oncogenic cells. Genes that may serve well in this scenario include costimulatory cytokines, such as genes that encode for GM-CSF, IL-2, and IL-12.

Other strategies would be to insert a gene into tumor cells to increase drug sensitivity. Various genes have been studied that include the insertion of thymidine kinase. Cells with this gene are sensitive to antiviral agents, such as acyclovir and ganciclovir, which are minimally to moderately cytotoxic to other host tissues. Alternative methods have been used to reduce patient toxicities to conventional drug therapy. This strategy has employed gene therapy in host cells that are given a drug resistance gene such as the P-glycoprotein or multiple drug resistant (MDR) gene.

Tumor Suppressor Gene Replacement

Another major cause of cancer involves dysfunction of tumor suppressor genes such as the *p53* and the retinoblastoma *(RB1)* genes. *p53* is a gene that has been found to arrest cellular replication and allow enough time for DNA repair. Damaged DNA not adequately repaired may lead to transcription of a mutated form of the wild type protein. The protein product, p53, has also been shown to induce cellular suicide of programmed cell death—apoptosis. Thus, the production of a mutated form of p53 may not be able to induce apoptosis leading to cell immortalization—a hallmark of tumor transformation. Therefore, a defect in *p53* expression can lead to uncontrolled growth regulation of damaged cells, which may introduce cellular transformation. By replacing the mutated *p53* gene with a wild-type *p53* gene, tumor suppression and replication attenuation was achieved in mice harboring human head, neck, and lung cancer cells.[15,16] Moreover, when cisplatin is combined with *p53* gene replacement therapy, initiation of the apoptotic process is noted. This, in turn, will induce further apoptosis, suggesting a synergistic reaction.[17]

Similarly, a defective *RB1* gene can lead to a loss of cellular control that eventually proceeds to retinal tumors and osteosarcomas. When a virus containing the wild-type *RB1* is inserted into murine lung and bladder cancer cells with a defective *RB1* gene, complete tumor suppression and tumor regression is seen. This illustrates how effectively replacing a tumor suppressor gene can efficiently eradicate certain types of cancer.

Immunotherapy

Insertion of Cytokine Gene

Besides targeting tumor-related genes, the genes involved in immune activation can also be an alternative gene therapy strategy. Insertion of immunogenic genes into tumors can increase an immune response against rapidly growing tumors. Early immunotherapy for cancer involves the insertion of the IL-2 gene. Using retroviral vectors to introduce the IL-2 gene into a weakly immunogenic methylcholanthrene-induced (CMS-5) tumor cells, CMS-5 expression of IL-2 showed an inverse correlation between IL-2 expression and tumor size. The results showed that tumor growth correlated inversely with the amount of IL-2 expressed and produced by the tumor cells. The same study also showed that mice immunized with IL-2-producing tumor cells are protected from a challenge with a highly tumorigenic dose of CMS-5 cells, suggesting the development of a specific and long-lasting immune response.[18]

Under the same principle, other cytokine genes can be inserted as well. A study using GM-CSF genes inserted into murine melanoma cells (B16) caused an increase in CD4+ and dendritic cells surrounding the tumor. Along with this result, approximately 40 percent of the transfected cells reject tumor cells after inoculation. These results implicate that immunotherapy can be used as an approach to induce tumor regression as well as a means of vaccination to prevent tumor formation.

Another approach for immunotherapy is the insertion of T-lymphocyte costimulatory gene into tumor cells to induce an immune response against tumor antigens. One such gene is the B7/BB1 gene, which encodes for a B7/BB1 antigen molecule on the APC that binds on to CD28 CTLA-4 receptors on the T-lymphocyte. The interaction between the B7/BB1 antigent molecule and the T-cell receptor leads to an increased production of IL-2, thereby costimulating the activation and expansion of CD8+ T-cells capable of killing tumors.[19]

Insertion of Tumor Rejection Antigen Gene

Tumor antigen epitopes can be incorporated into vectors as a way to increase immune response against the tumor. One study involving the transfer of human carcinoembryonic antigen (CEA) gene in mouse adenocarcinoma cells found that the threshold dose of 50 μg of CEA polynucleotide plasmid is capable of inducing CEA specific lymphoblastic transformation, lymphokine release, and antibody response. In addition, as early as three weeks after the first vaccination, sufficient anti-CEA antibody is generated in mice to protect against syngeneic CEA-expressing colon carcinoma cells.[20] Another study utilizing DNA liposomal human leukocyte antigen-B7 (HLA-B7) gene in human melanoma cells showed an increase in tumor-specific cytotoxic T-lymphocytes and regression of cutaneous nodules. These studies reinforce the concept that gene therapy can be used as a vaccine to stimulate immune response against tumors.

Insertion of Antisense RNA Gene

Unfortunately, not all tumor cells respond equivalently to this therapy. This may be due to the following reasons: the heterogeneous expression of antigen on tumor cells, the defects in antigen presentation in tumor cells, and the factors produced by cancer cells to suppress antigen presentation. One of the factors that is highly expressed in glioblastoma and breast cancers is the insulin-like growth factor (IGF-I). Expression of IGF-I allows tumor cells to evade detection by the immune system. Thus, another strategy of cancer gene therapy involves the transfer of antisense IGF-I RNA gene to block gene expression. A study transferring the IGF-I antisense gene into rat glioblastoma showed an increase in CD8+ lymphocyte expansion, which correlates to the observed tumor regression, complete loss of tumorgenicity for 13 months, and prevention of tumor formation by nontransfected cells.[21] This study suggests that antisense RNA gene therapy can indirectly stimulate the immune response against cancer.

Insertion of Drug-Resistant Gene

In addition to the activation of the immune response against tumors, cancer gene therapy can also be used as a means to enhance the pharmacological effects of chemotherapy. This can be accomplished by the insertion of drug-resistant genes that enhance bone marrow protection during chemotherapy. This would allow higher doses of a chemotherapeutic agent to be given with less toxicity and more efficacy. The bone marrow of mice after receiving the multidrug-resistance gene (MDR1) conferred resistance to the myelosuppressive effects of chemotherapeutic agents such as doxorubicin, daunomycin, paclitaxel, vinblastine, vincristine, etoposide, and actinomycin D.

A later study utilizing a retroviral gene transfer of a different drug-resistance gene, the multidrug-resistance protein gene (MRP), found parallel bone marrow resistance to doxorubicin and vincristine. Interestingly enough, the drug-resistant effect of the MRP gene is poorly reversed by MDR1 reversal drugs, namely cyclosporin-A and verapamil. Therefore, this MRP gene therapy can be used synergistically with MDR1 reversal drugs to decrease the MDR1 expression in tumors while maintaining the hematopoietic protective effect in the bone marrow.

A third drug-resistant gene studied is the gene encoding the enzyme dihydrofolate reductase (DHFR), which is involved in the biosynthesis of purines, thymidylate, and glycine. The chemotherapeutic agent methotrexate (MTX) exerts its effect by competitively inhibiting DHFR. Therefore, besides killing tumor cells, MTX therapy is also toxic to other rapidly proliferating cells in the body such as the bone marrow and gastrointestinal mucosal cells. A study involving the transplantation of the DHFR gene into the bone marrow of mice demonstrated protection from hematopoietic and gastrointestinal toxicity effects from low and lethal doses of MTX.[22] Thus, this approach allows higher doses of chemotherapeutic agents to be administered to the patients with less toxic effects.

Insertion of Drug-Sensitivity Gene

Another gene that can be inserted to augment the specificity and targeting effects of chemotherapeutic agents is the drug-sensitivity gene. The prototype gene transfer involves the use of herpes simplex virus thymidine kinase gene *(HSV-tk)* along with the administration of ganciclovir (GCV) for the treatment of gliomas. In order for GCV to be active inside the cell, it must be triphosphorylated by thymidine kinase. A study was performed by Culver and colleagues in which the *HSV-tk*-containing retroviral vector was transferred into rat glioma cells.[23] Five days posttransduction, these cells were treated with systemic GCV. Theoretically, cells that are transduced should become sensitive to GCV treatment. In fact, rapid and complete tumor regression was achieved with the retroviral-transduced cells.

In the same study, cells that were not transduced by the *HSV-tk* gene were also killed. This is called the bystander effect, which is possibly mediated by the following mechanisms: the transfer of toxic metabolic products of GCV through gap junctions, the transfer of hydrolases or other enzymes triggered by apoptosis of nearby cells, or the induction of an immune response against the tumor through a priming effect. A study focusing on the bystander effect showed that 10 percent *HSV-tk*-positive tumor cells will lead to the eradication of a majority of tumor cells while 50 percent of *HSV-tk*-positive tumor cells will lead to complete tumor regression.[24] These studies suggest that the use of the drug-sensitivity gene confers the advantages of enhancing cell-specific cytotoxicity by inducing a powerful bystander effect which allows cells surrounding the tumor cells to be eradicated.

CLINICAL TRIALS WITH GENE THERAPY

Cystic Fibrosis

Cystic fibrosis is a fatal hereditary disease that results from mutation of the cystic fibrosis transmembrane conduction regulator (CFTR) gene. A defect in this gene results due to deletion of a phenylalanine residue from its polypeptide backbone at position 1480. The CFTR gene product is a cyclic-AMP regulated protein that controls chloride efflux across the epithelial cell membrane.

This autosomal recessive genetic disorder affects one in 250,000 Caucasians in the United States. In cystic fibrosis, the production of abnormal mucus can cause obstruction of glands and ducts in various organs, particularly respiratory airways. Blockade of ducts and glands can lead to tissue damage resulting in cellular lysis. The increased concentration of DNA will increase the viscosity of mucus in the airways, culminating in increased risk of bronchitis, pneumonia, ateletcasis, and parenchymal scarring. Patients with advanced disease can develop pneumothorax and cor pulmonale, which are poor prognostic factors for survival. Current treatments focus on ameliorating the symptomatic disease, where antibiotics are instituted for infectious complications. Dornase (DNase) is administered to reduce the viscosity of the sputum in affected patients.

A full-length cDNA encoding for CFTR gene was cloned into a retroviral vector. Cells without functional CFTR gene infected with the transformed retroviral vector had normal chloride efflux in response to adenylate cyclase stimulation. The anion efflux of the transfected epithelium was functionally comparable to that of normal tracheal epithelial cells. This study suggested that gene therapy for cystic fibrosis using aerosolized CFTR-positive retroviruses might provide a cure for this deadly disease.[11]

In another study, the cystic fibrosis transmembrane conduction reductase gene (CFTR) was inserted into lung epithelia using adenovirus vectors.[25] However, the viruses were introduced into the body via inhalation, where the vectors were nebulized and inhaled. Patients who took part in the study had detectable levels of CFTR in the cells. Unfortunately, it was discovered that adenoviral vectors are able to elicit an undesirable immune response, thus repeated administration of adenoviral vectors is prohibited. Another potential problem associated with using adenovirus is that the vector may regain replication competency. This occurs when the virus is able to reacquire the ability to replicate through homologous recombination with the wild-type adenovirus found in the body.

CONCLUSION

Gene therapy is still in its pioneer stages of development. Many in vivo and ex vivo studies have shown that gene therapy can be efficacious and safe under controlled conditions (see Table 7.5). In the past decade, there have been major advances in gene therapy, especially in the area of cancer therapy. Most of these advances depend on a basic

TABLE 7.5. Human Gene Therapy Protocols (Ex Vivo)

Gene	Target Cell	Disease
Adenosine deaminase (ADA)	Peripheral T-lymphocytes	ADA deficiency
β-Glucocerebrodidase	CD34+ lymphocytes	Gaucher's disease
Tumor necrosis factor (TNF)	Tumor-infiltrating lympho-cytes	Malignant melanoma
Tumor necrosis factor (TNF)	Tumor cells	Advanced tumor
Interleukin-2 (IL-2)	Tumor cells	Advanced tumor
Interleukin-4	Tumor cells	Renal cell carcinoma
Inteferon-γ	Melanoma cells	Melanoma
Human LDL receptor	Liver cells	High cholesterol
Factor IX	Skin fibroblasts	Hemophilia B
MLR-1	Bone marrow cells	Cancer

understanding of human genetics and molecular biology. The ongoing clinical trials today will help determine the optimal gene delivery system and conditions for future gene therapy protocols. The future challenge is to design vectors that have an increased efficiency of gene expression and an increased precision in cell targeting, which will advance the final clinical outcome for the patients. All in all, gene therapy is an emerging medical therapy that offers promising clinical cures in the future.

NOTES

1. Putnam D. Antisense strategies and therapeutic applications. *Am J Health Sys Pharm* 1996;53(2):151-160.

2. Mol J, Van Der Krol A (Eds). Antisense oligonucleotides. Antisense nucleic acids and proteins. New York: Marcel Dekker, Inc., 1991, pp. 47-93.

3. Askari F, McDonnell W. Antisense-oligonucleotide therapy. *New Engl J Med* 1996;334(5):316-318.

4. Azad RF, Driver VB, Tanaka K, Crooke RM, Anderson KP. Antiviral activity of a phosphorothioate oligonucleotide complementary to RNA of the human cytomegalovirus major immediate-early region. *Antimic Agents and Chemoth* 1993; 37(9):1945-1954.

5. Jacobson MA. Treatment of cytomegalovirus retinitis in patients with the acquired immunodeficiency syndrome. *Drug Ther* 1997;337(2):105-114.

6. Hoover DR, Graham NM, Bacellar H, Murphy R, Visscher B, Anderson R, McArthur J. An epidemiologic analysis of *Mycobacterium avium* complex disease in homosexual men infected with human immunodeficiency virus type 1. *Clin Infect Dis* 1995;20(5):1250-1258.

7. Product Information: Vitravene, Fomivirsen. Isis Pharmaceuticals, Carlsbad, CA, 1998.

8. Mirabelli CK, Bennett CF, Anderson K, Crooke ST. In vitro and in vivo pharmacologic activities of antisense oligonucleotides. *Anti-Cancer Drug Design* 1991; 6:647-661.

9. Zhang Y, Mukhopadhyay L. Retroviral vector-mediated transduction of K-*ras* antisense RNA into human lung cancer cells inhibits expression of the malignant phenotype. *Hum Gene Ther* 1993;4:451-460.

10. Feng M, Cabrera G, Deshane J, Scanlon KJ, Curiel DT. Neoplastic reversion accomplished by high efficiency adenoviral-mediated delivery of an anti-*ras* ribozyme. *Cancer Res* 1995;55:2024-2028.

11. Crystal RG, Jaffe A, Brody S, Mastrangeli A, McElvaney NG, Rosenfeld M, Chu CS, Danel C, Hay J, Eissa T. A phase 1 study, in cystic fibrosis patients, of the safety, toxicity, and biological efficacy of a single administration of a replication deficient, recombinant adenovirus carrying the cDNA of the normal cystic fibrosis transmembrane conductance regulator gene in the lung. *Human Gene Ther* 1995; 6(5):643-666.

12. Ali M, Lemoine N, Ring C. The use of DNA viruses as vectors for gene therapy. *Gene Ther* 1994;1:367-384.

13. Mastrangelo M, Berd D, Nathan F, Lattime E. Gene therapy for human cancer: An essay for clinicians. *Semin Oncol* 1996;23(1):4-21.

14. Wolff JA, Malone RW, Williams P, Chong W, Ascadi G, Jani A, Felgner PL. Direct gene transfer into mouse muscle in vivo. *Science* 1990;247(4949 Pt 1):1465-1468.

15. Liu TJ, Zhang WW, Taylor DL, Roth JA, Goepfert H, Clayman GL. Growth suppression of human head and neck cancer cells by the introduction of a wild-type *p53* gene via a recombinant adenovirus. *Cancer Res* 1994;54:3662-3667.

16. Fujiwara T, Cai DW, Georges RN, Mukhopadhyay T, Grimm EA, Roth JA. Therapeutic effect of a retroviral wild-type *p53* expression vector in an orthotopic lung cancer model. *J Natl Cancer Inst* 1994;86(19):1458-1462.

17. Fujiwara T, Grimm EA, Mukhopadhyay T, Zhang WW, Owen-Schaub LB, Roth JA. Induction of chemosensitivity in human lung cancer cells in vivo by adenovirus-mediated transfer of the wild-type *p53* gene. *Cancer Res* 1994;54:2287-2291.

18. Gansbacher B, Zier K, Daniels B, Cronin K, Bannerji R, Gilboa E. Interleukin 2 gene transfer into tumor cells abrogates tumorgenicity and induces protective immunity. *J Exp Med* 1990;172:1217-1224.

19. Schwartz R. Costimulation of T-lymphocytes: The role of CD28, CTLA-4, and B7/BB1 in Interleukin-2 production and immunotherapy. *Cell* 1992;71:1065-1068.

20. Conry RM, LoBuglio AF, Loechel F, Moore SE, Sumerel LA, Barlow DL, Curiel DT. A carcinoembryonic antigen polynucleotide vaccine has in vivo antitumor activity. *Gene Ther* 1995;2:59-65.

21. Trojan J, Johnson TR, Rudin SD, Ilan J, Tykocinski ML, Ilan J. Treatment and prevention of rat glioblastomas by immunogenic C6 cells expressing antisense insulin-like growth factor I RNA. *Science* 1993;259:94-101.

22. May C, Gunther R, Mclvor RS. Protection of mice from lethal doses of Methotrexate by transplantation with transgenic marrow expressing drug-resistant dihydrofolate reductase activity. *Blood* 1995;86(6):2439-2448.

23. Culver KW, Ram Z, Wallbridge S, Ishii H, Oldfield EH, Blaese RM. In vivo gene transfer with retroviral vector-producer cells for treatment of experimental brain tumors [comment]. *Science* 1992;256(5063):1550-1552.

24. Freeman SM, Abboud CN, Whartenby KA, Packman CH, Koeplin DS, Moolten FL, Abraham GN. The bystander effect: Tumor regression when a fraction of the tumor mass is genetically modified. *Cancer Res* 1993;53:5274-5283.

25. Crystal RG, McElvaney NG, Rosenfeld MA, Chu CS, Mastrangeli A, Hay JG, Brody SL, Jaffe HA, Eissa NT, Danel C. Administration of an adenovirus containing the human CFTR cDNA to the respiratory tract of individuals with cystic fibrosis [comment]. *Nature Genetics* 1994;8(1):42-51.

Index

Page numbers followed by the letter "b" indicate boxed material; those followed by the letter "f" indicate a figure; and those followed by the letter "t" indicate a table.

186 *HANDBOOK OF PHARMACEUTICAL BIOTECHNOLOGY*

Antihemophilic Factor (Recombinate™)
(rAHF) *(continued)*
clinical trials, 51-52
dosage and administration, 51-52,
53t
pharmacokinetics, 51
pharmacology, 50-51
preparation and storage, 52
Antisense RNA gene insertion, for
cancer, 179
Antisense therapy, 162, 163, 164
cancers, 179
ras oncognes, 166-167
Arterial thrombosis formation, 66
ASSENT-2, AMI trial, 78
Atherectomy, 17

ß-thalassemia, 161
Baby hamster kidney (BHK) cells, 53
Bacteria, as host cell, 6-7
Bacterial plasmids, 2-4
insertion, 3f
Ballistic DNA injection, 173t, 174
Basiliximab (Simulect®), 26-29
adverse reactions, 30
clinical trials, 28-29
dosage and administration, 28
pharmacokinetics, 27-28
product information, 27
Becaplermin (Regranex®), 135-137
adverse reactions, 136
clinical trials, 135-136
dosage and administration, 136-137
pharmacokinetics, 135
product information, 135
Biological agent production, 7-9
Biotechnology, definition, 1
Bloodborn disease, and hemophilia
treatment, 45, 46
Bone marrow transplantation (BMT),
21, 65
rhGM-CSF trials, 126-127
Breast cancer, 35, 36-37
Bronchopulmonary dysplasia (BPD), 39

Cachectin, and TNF, 146
Cadaveric liver allografts, 29

Calcium salt complexation, 4, 6
Cancer gene therapy, 176-181
Chemotherapy-induced neutropenia,
120, 124
Chimerization process, 11-12, 13f
Chinese hamster ovary (CHO) cells, 7
Chloride transport receptor (CTFR), 79
Christmas disease (Type B
hemophilia), 43
Chronic granulomatous disease (CGD),
112
IFN-γ 1b clinical trials, 114-115
Chronic hepatitis B, 101-102
Chronic hepatitis C, 102
Chronic pancreatic insufficiency, 65
Chronic renal failure (CRF)
anemia treatment, 130
rhEPO clinical trials, 131
Class I and II CSFs, 118
Coagulation cascade, 43, 44b
Colony-stimulating factors (CSFs),
117-118
Complementary DNA (cDNA), 6, 8, 9,
169
Condylomata acuminata, 96
Crick, Francis, 1
Crohn's Disease (CD), 153-154
Infliximab trials, 155-156
Cyclophosphamide, doxorubicin,
dexamethasone (CAD), 103
Cyclophosphamide, doxorubicin,
etoposide (CAE), 121
Cystic fibrosis (CF), 78-79, 161
gene therapy trials, 181-182
Cytokine gene insertion, for cancer,
177-178
Cytokine release syndrome (CRS), 25
risk characteristics, 27b
Cytokines, definitions, 85, 141
Cytomegalovirus (CMV), 88
retinitis, 163-164
Cytotoxic T-Lymphocytes (CTLs), 85,
87, 95

Daclizumab (Zenapax®), 29-31
adverse reactions, 31, 32t
clinical trials, 30-31
dosage and administration, 30
pharmacokinetics, 30
product information, 29-30